Super

'Christopher Dines has used his ow~ ....
teaching. He has demonstrated e ....oming
challenges which he shares with his ʳᵉᵃᵈers and listeners as a means of
joining them in their own. His kind and soothing voice, combined with
excellent examples of ideas to help calm the mind and body, practice
self-care and move through obstacles, is inspiring. I recommend his book
Super Self-Care without reservation.'

Eileen Rockefeller, author, venture philanthropist (USA)

'*Super Self-Care* is of a sacred safe space—the divine within you and me.
Christopher Dines gets it, and writes of it, at the deepest level. Find in this
book a high calling inward, to do good to yourself, to gear up for beautiful
relationships, and a great life onward.'

Michael Cogdill, American journalist, anchor,
novelist, screenwriter, and film producer

'*Super Self-Care* is as comprehensive as it is illuminating. Christopher writes
about a form of self-care that is leagues beyond the buzz-wordy clichés
that a lot of us are inundated with by advertising, which tend to focus on
buying one's way into fulfilment. In many ways, *Super Self-Care* is about
radical new ways to parent yourself and give birth to the beautiful being
who lives within you—even though his or her wings might have been
clipped by anything from toxic relationships, to addiction, to the wear and
tear we suffer at the hands of limiting beliefs and habits that don't serve us.'

Kelly McNelis, founder of Women for One and
author of *Your Messy Brilliance*

'Christopher Dines' book, *Super Self-Care* provides important spiritual tools,
which will assist you to create a more fulfilling and authentic life.'

Christine Handy, motivational speaker and best selling
author of *Walk Beside Me*

Super Self-Care

How to find lasting freedom from addiction, toxic relationships and dysfunctional lifestyles

CHRISTOPHER DINES

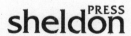
sheldon PRESS

First published by Sheldon Press in 2020

An imprint of John Murray Press

An Hachette UK company

1

A CIP catalogue record for this title is available from the British Library

Trade Paperback ISBN 978 152933 054 0

eBook ISBN 978 152933 070 0

Typeset by Cenveo® Publisher Services.

John Murray Press policy is to use papers that are natural, renewable and recyclable products and made from wood grown in sustainable forests. The logging and manufacturing processes are expected to conform to the environmental regulations of the country of origin.

Sheldon Press
Carmelite House
50 Victoria Embankment
London EC4Y 0DZ

www.sheldonpress.co.uk

Printed and bound in Great Britain by Clays Ltd, Elcograf S.p.A.

This book is dedicated to Mary McGahan.

Contents

Acknowledgements

I would like to thank Victoria Roddam at Hodder & Stoughton for playing a major role in the publishing of this book: her hard work, professionalism and encouragement have been invaluable. Thanks, too, to Zakirah Alam and everyone involved at Sheldon Press.

Thanks are also due to Kelly McNelis for writing a heartfelt foreword and for her continued support in the USA; Eileen Rockefeller Growald for her endorsement and encouragement over the years; James Alexander for creating a space for me to share my ideas and for his invaluable feedback; Edward M. Frazer for encouraging me to pursue my goals, and Mary McGahan for looking over an early draft of this book. Many thanks to Christine Handy for endorsing my book; I appreciate your support. Thank you to Michael Cogdill for supporting "Super Self-Care", and for encouraging me to write in my early 20s.

Finally, I would like to thank you, the reader, for investing your time into reading this book. Many, many thanks.

About the author

Christopher Dines is a British mindfulness teacher and writer. He has published eight books and facilitated workshops, seminars, retreats, school talks and corporate events, assisting people to reduce stress and enhance their emotional wellbeing and serenity.

Foreword

When my friend Christopher Dines sent me a copy of his new book, *Super Self-Care: How to find lasting freedom from addiction, toxic relationships and dysfunctional lifestyles*, I was sold on the title alone. As the founder of a global community that's all about moving into collective resilience and power, no matter the odds that are stacked against us, I am all about the practical tools that will help us to live our best lives.

Then, as I got deeper into the book, my enthusiasm grew. I thought to myself, Finally! A book that doesn't pay lip service to self-care but actually talks about the whys and the hows in depth!

Super Self-Care is as comprehensive as it is illuminating. Christopher writes about a form of self-care that is leagues beyond the buzz-wordy clichés that a lot of us are inundated with by advertising, which tend to focus on buying one's way into fulfilment. In many ways, *Super Self-Care* is about radical new ways to parent yourself and give birth to the beautiful being who lives within you – even though your wings might have been clipped by anything from toxic relationships, to addiction, to the wear and tear you have suffered at the hands of limiting beliefs and habits that don't serve you.

For years, I've led retreats that help women claim their voices and their 'messy brilliance' (which I define as the polished gem of our truth and beauty, which we discover only by diving into the mess and the so-called darkness). As an incest survivor and someone who's suffered my fair share of hardships, I know what it's like to walk through the muck and feel buried beneath the weight of it all. But as a mother, author and teacher, I also understand that our trauma and pain can be potent fuel for transformation. They can be the very things that equip us with empathy, perspective, wisdom and compassion for ourselves and others. They can also be the very ingredients that lead us to lasting joy and peace – the kind that cannot be taken away from us, no matter what challenges we're facing in our lives.

This brilliant observation that it is our 'brokenness' that has the power to lead us back to our essential wholeness is at the heart of Christopher's book.

I know Christopher Dines as a friend, colleague and one of the Truthtellers in my global community, Women For One. Christopher has repeatedly shared his wisdom with my community; he has written and talked about the power of kindness in moving through addiction and recovery, as well as what it means to cultivate authentic self-acceptance in the face of paralysing shame.

Christopher is someone whom I deeply respect, because he is a man who walks his talk. He's also a kindred spirit who has gone through the school of hard knocks and come out a better person for it.

Self-care is an ongoing process, and we need reliable and credible guides to help us navigate the way. In *Super Self-Care*, Christopher takes you on a journey through the physical, emotional, mental and spiritual value of self-care, and how you can pick yourself up and sustain the courage and faith to keep going – especially when you face setbacks or doubt your ability to rise above your circumstances.

Gentleness is at the core of Christopher's message. His focus on the power of vulnerability, the importance of asking for help and finding support on the self-care path, and removing yourself from the clutches of shame are all aspects I seldom hear self-care experts talk about. Christopher also offers gorgeous insight on dealing with resistance and limiting beliefs, gaining awareness of dysfunctional patterns that have been with you since childhood, and honouring your feelings while learning to locate the still point in the centre of inner tumult. All of this is powerful food for thought that will support you throughout the book.

In this book, you'll find everything from powerful personal anecdotes to inspiring activities and guided meditations that will help you put the concepts in each chapter into practice. And, of course, you'll also get plenty of timeless wisdom that will allow you to embrace your whole self. The questions in each chapter will guide you through a deep process of self-inquiry that will be foundational when it comes to creating your own unique self-care rituals.

Ultimately, in the most non-shaming way possible, Christopher is here to help you gain awareness of the patterns that keep you feeling stuck or in a place of despair and hopelessness. But, as he shares, 'rock bottom' doesn't have to be a life sentence. As Christopher skilfully reveals, self-care isn't an all-or-nothing journey. We can all find joy in the midst of pain, comfort in the wake of loss, and awareness right in the heart of chaos.

Super Self-Care is a book that is gentle, like its author, but packed with powerful methods for finding peace, and ultimately the kind of freedom that we are all searching for. Although the current state of our inner and outer worlds can feel overwhelming to sit with, Christopher demonstrates that it's possible to do so with courage, humour, commitment and deep self-love.

Every single one of us is here to become who we were always meant to be: powerful, purposeful beings capable of transforming our lives and worlds for the better. As the old saying goes, we are the ones we've been waiting for. *Super Self-Care* will make that sense of coming home to yourself all the sweeter.

Kelly McNelis, founder of Women For One (USA) and author of Your Messy Brilliance

Introduction: What is super self-care?

A great many people still struggle with the idea of self-care and will dismiss the idea of prioritizing their own wellbeing as somehow being selfish. Some of these people may have been conditioned from a very young age to put others' needs before their own in order to serve the greater good. They may question the idea that it would be better for society as a whole if we all made our own wellbeing (mental, emotional, physical, spiritual, financial and social) a priority.

While placing others' needs before your own might appear to be morally sound, in reality it can bring in its wake burnout, jealousy, resentment and confusion. Self-care is often confused with selfishness or self-centredness. For many years I did exactly this. I abandoned my own wellbeing by putting the needs of others before mine and the consequences were very detrimental.

The definition of self-centredness in the *Oxford English Dictionary* is: 'The tendency to think only about yourself and not about the needs or feelings of other people.' The fact is self-care is the complete opposite of self-centredness. The concept of self-care is most definitely a worthy ideal. Healthy relationships and improving mental, emotional, spiritual and financial wellbeing will help us to live joyfully, serenely and prosperously, which will lead to us being much better placed to serve others.

Rather than existing in survival mode, we can make a decision to do things differently and truly thrive. This is my definition of super self-care. Many people are indeed practising super self-care in their lives. Their wellbeing is a priority, and they make no bones about this.

In order to thrive in this world and have fulfilling relationships we have to be authentic and honest with ourselves. Are we living a healthy and fulfilling life or are we still in denial about feeling stuck? Are we wrapped up in co-dependent behaviour? Are we taking care of our bodies or are we playing out an unconscious script – subconscious patterns of behaviour formed while we were children from decades ago? How can we care for others if we do not care for ourselves? How can we teach a child to love him or herself if we cannot demonstrate self-love? How can we love our family and friends if we do not love ourselves? We have to *be* before we can *do*.

Naturally, there will be some people who scoff at the idea of super self-care. There are many who are so unaware of their own self-loathing and self-destructive behaviour that they will not be able to tune in to the concept of super self-care, because it is completely at odds with their lifestyle. They might need to hit a serious rock bottom before they will examine their own lives. In my case, I had to hit rock bottom aged 21 before I could listen to those who had previously encouraged me to take care of myself. I will share my experience on this matter in the following chapters.

Humanness

The power of listening to others and reflecting on one's own belief system can work tremendously well for those of us in recovery. While leading my 'Super Self-Care' seminar, in Bond Street, London, I observed my clients sharing their experiences regarding love, recovery, self-compassion and long-term committed romantic relationships, professional relationships, family dynamics and freedom from addictive behaviours. My clients sat around a large table with a notepad and a pen, while I asked them a series of questions such as: 'What does love mean to you?', 'How are you getting on in your recovery from co-dependency and addictive behaviours?', 'What does super self-care mean to you?' 'How do you practise self-love in your everyday life?,' 'How often do you deliberately use your imagination to rewire your brain?' and 'Is the emotion of fear paralysing your efforts to have loving relationships?'

I asked my clients to share their answers without giving out unsolicited advice to other participants. It was amazing to see the group courageously share their ideas. I occasionally shared my own personal experience and factual data I had collected on the subject of super self-care, as a result of my work as a mindfulness teacher and writer. However, it was important for the group to find their own identity.

After one hour, as a result of personal boundaries being put in place, the individuals felt safe enough to gently give non-shaming feedback to each other, based on their own experience. They demonstrated courage, vulnerability and a desire to grow. I walked away from the seminar and understood more deeply how personal and collective boundaries can create a suitable environment to have meaningful, authentic and safe conversations. Prior to this seminar, I had led over 150 private seminars for both companies and self-referrals, but the depth and substance at this seminar was different. Such was my enthusiasm that I decided to write this book, *Super Self-Care*.

I can see now that the last 15 years of my life have been a gradual process of practising super self-care, which started the day I got sober in recovery. I am recovering from drug and alcohol addiction, co-dependency, love addiction, compulsive hiding and severe trauma. I stopped drinking aged 21 and have steadily made progress in my own recovery. I have not drunk alcohol or taken drugs for close to 15 years. My recovery has not been a straight line; there have been many twists and turns, but nonetheless progress has been made. I have been working in the addictions and personal development fields for over 13 years, both in drug and alcohol rehabs and private corporations. I have spent my entire adult life assisting people both personally and professionally to practise super self-care.

Most of us are searching for love, trust, courage, confidence, validation, intimacy, serenity, success and acceptance from our family, friends and fellow professionals. Having evaluated my own journey and observed many people I have spent time with, I have come to realize that we already have inside of us what we are searching for. We have a brain which we can use to change our behaviour and demonstrate equanimity. We have a mind which we can use to direct our brain to reduce low-grade chronic stress and produce calm. We can learn to monitor our thoughts, discard limiting beliefs, and get in touch with our feelings. We have a body which enables us to connect and integrate with our fellow humans beings. This is possible, right now, in this very moment.

As a result of having a mind, brain and body, we can build healthy, non-shaming relationships. We can learn to create relationships which are based on trust and authenticity, rather than fear, co-dependency and control. We can heal our emotional wounds (our frozen pain which stifles our emotional, spiritual and physical development) and relearn to trust ourselves and others again. As a result of healing our frozen emotional pain, we can be in a long-term committed, erotic loving relationship. We can discard our masks, survival behavioural traits and let go of our false self – thereby accessing our true self. Authenticity is possible in recovery. Love and trust are possible to realize in recovery. Financial recovery is possible in recovery. I have personally experienced this, and I can think of several hundred people I know personally who have also realized this, too. Millions more people around the world are rebuilding their lives, one day at a time.

How to make the most of this book

I have based this book on my personal and professional experience (and on many years of in-depth research), to assist you to explore different ways to practise super self-care in your own life. Authenticity is a constant theme in this book. Once you begin to unlearn your past conditioning and can discard disempowering ideas about *who you are*, your reality will begin to change at once.

We will uncover the many reasons which cause us to feel stuck in our lives. We will explore different ways to transcend our subconscious levels of awareness, shame and co-dependency. We will uncover the importance of gentleness and vulnerability, and how we can use authenticity to enhance our emotional and spiritual lives. We will explore creating nourishing relationships, professional, romantic and personal, and love. Love is truly a mystery, which transcends reason. In my view, love is the bedrock of recovery from all addictive behaviours. Love is a healing energy which already dwells in our hearts.

Lastly, I have created an abundance of exercises in Chapter 6: Creating new goals and changing your behaviour. I highly recommend approaching the final chapter with another person. By and large, it is extremely difficult to manifest our desires and change behaviours without having a sufficient support system and infrastructure. Old ingrained habits will be too difficult to transcend for most people who attempt to evolve without human assistance. In Chapter 6, we will take a look at imagination. We can use our imagination to visualize a better reality for us to live in. Our imagination is an amazing mental faculty in the prefrontal cortex, which we can draw upon to see our future selves living peacefully and abundantly. We can emotionally connect with our imagination, therefore having an impact on our behaviour. Once we are emotionally in sync with our imagination, we can act accordingly and literally change the way we live.

I have created guided scripted meditations, imagination exercises and provided tools to enhance your emotional and spiritual recovery. You will need a pen and a notebook (use this notebook specifically for your super self-care practice).

Please write by hand, not on your computer, tablet or smart-phone. You can connect more deeply with your *feelings* when you are writing on a piece of paper. *Super Self-Care* is about thriving, one day at a time. *Super Self-Care* is a solution-based book. Take your time going through the exercises and discuss these ideas with someone you know who is serious about thriving in life.

Treat this book like a thorough, honest, self-appraisal

This book is really a gentle, non-shaming, self-appraisal. There are 147 questions to answer, and the self-appraisal has been written in such a way to draw your attention to your strengths and areas in your life which require a slight adjustment. The book has been written in such a way as to communicate at a deep feeling level of awareness.

If you answer all of the questions in this book and discuss all of your answers with a non-shaming person in recovery consciously seeking to improve their life, I can guarantee you that you will expand your self-awareness. What you choose to do with your new self-awareness is entirely up to you. The final chapter works as a guide to help you visualize and use your imagination to channel your awareness to create a new goal, such as enhancing your relationships. Through meditation, visualization and meditation, you can expand your life and enhance your relationships.

1

Being aware of your subconscious feelings and behaviours

> The degree to which a person can grow is directly proportional to the amount of truth he can accept about himself without running away.
>
> *Leland Val Van De Wall*

Many of us feel stuck in our lives. This can certainly feel like a lonely existence where we are often dominated by frustration, depression and, sometimes, rage. Some people struggle with building a fulfilling career, while others find it hard to earn enough money to meet their financial responsibilities, let alone their wants. Some people believe it is impossible to have long-term, committed, romantic relationships, while others struggle to maintain friendships. Many people are hurting while caring for loved ones and often find the responsibility all too overwhelming because they believe there is no way out. Feeling lost in life often occurs when we feel stuck and unable to progress. Feeling lost is often a symptom of isolation, unresolved grief and a lack of presence-awareness. Uncertainty, confusion, shame and excessive guilt often drive a sense of feeling lost.

Feeling baffled by our results in life

Many of us earnestly try to build healthy and functional relationships with ourselves and others, only to find ourselves *feeling stuck* in a cycle of disappointment, frustration and despair. We tried so hard to determine our destiny, but ended up producing similar outcomes and results year after year. Some of us tried to have loving romantic relationships but failed miserably. We tried to build a fulfilling and prosperous career and friendly professional relationships, only to create the exact opposite. We tried so hard to practise self-care but there was something deep within us which triggered us to demonstrate self-neglect. When we tried to rationally and consciously examine why we were making very little progress in a particular area of our lives, our thinking became hazy. *We could not philosophize or psychologize our way out of feeling baffled by the disappointing results in our lives.*

Some of us read hundreds of self-help books, attended meditation retreats and went to see a professional regarding mental and emotional health problems, only to make modest progress at best. How can this be? It is almost as though our lives have been predetermined for us by some other unknown factor, which we could not circumvent despite our best efforts to do so. The sad fact is that many of us stop attempting to improve our lives after many unsuccessful attempts and drift back into a deep hypnotic, subconscious trance. We go back into survival mode and gravitate towards those who resonate energetically with our own subconscious programming.

Something inside you is often working in opposition to your goals

Why is that all too often when a person declares that she wants to change her life, within a matter of months she has given up her declaration entirely? Why is it that when a person states that he wants to get physically fit, his intention fizzles out within weeks? Why do many people say that they are willing to work on themselves so that they can have a loving, committed romantic relationship, only to find themselves behaving in ways which destroy trust, commitment and engagement? Why do millions of highly intelligent people decide that they are going to improve their relationships, but their behaviour states otherwise? Why is the mental faculty of reason alone, unable to change the way a person behaves? Have we not been taught in most of our education institutions that we can rationalize our way out of our problems?

Having been a mindfulness teacher for over 13 years, and practised mindfulness in my personal life, I have come to realize that, although the faculty of reason is important, it alone cannot change our behaviour. I spent years believing that gathering information with respect to how to change my life would help me to change my behaviour. It did no such thing. This was a hard lesson to learn; reason and the intellect can play only a very modest part in changing our behaviour. Granted, we need good information but only for the purpose of utilizing such information. Through utilizing the prefrontal cortex, which is responsible for reason, logic, empathy, imagination, compassion and creativity, we may well have *imagined* ourselves having fulfilling relationships; however, such an image was of very little use because we could not emotionally and physically connect with our vision. Our vision of ourselves having fulfilling relationships produced zero results because we were consumed with fear.

The problem is that many of us rely on our everyday, repetitive, mundane thought-life (which is mostly memory), and neglect to monitor our emotions and feelings. This is what keeps us feeling trapped, and therefore stops us from behaving differently towards making positive changes in our lives. We consciously say we want to do something, but *feel* at odds with what we have declared we wish to do. We *think* we want to change, but we *feel* otherwise. How baffling! The deep feelings we have, which we can detect by mindfully paying attention to our body, is what we call our subconscious programming. Such subjective programming is what determines how we behave most of time.

Remember the resistance you felt when you decided to change an ingrained habit? You could physically feel the resistance, anxiety and fear throughout your entire body. You might have felt physically drained while attempting to change a habit, as a result of your tempestuous emotional state. This was your subconscious programming operating in your body. Your limbic system and brainstem went into overdrive, and therefore your body felt threatened by your attempt to change its regular patterns of behaviour. For instance, we have known for some time that memories and emotions are stored in the tissues in the human body. The human body remembers every thought, feeling, sensation and experience impressed on it. Since we were in our mother's womb and thereafter, the body has registered every emotional experience. Frozen grief, trauma, and all feelings and sensations are stored as memory banks in the human body. Thus the saying, *the body never lies*.

The human body is where we can access our subconscious programming, by being aware of our emotions. If we say we want to learn a new language but *feel* like we cannot, our subconscious programming will therefore produce all sorts of reasons why we cannot learn a new language. To challenge these excuses will be difficult at first, until we can reprogram me the emotional layers of resistance towards learning a new language. A guide to changing our subconscious programming and practising self-directed neuroplasticity can be found in Chapter 6: Creating new goals and changing your behaviour.

While I was writing this chapter, my partner reminded me that I still have three different types of fresh loose leaf tea to drink. I have an ingrained habit of usually making a pot of tea using tea bags and letting the tea bags brew in a teapot. There is something within me that *feels* that it takes too long to make a pot using fresh tea and that there is an inconvenience in using a strainer to stop the tea leaves spilling into the cup. I decided to get up and make a pot of tea using loose leaf tea, after my partner pointed this out to me, just to challenge my habit. This is a rather mundane example of how my habits can stop me from doing something which I would otherwise enjoy and benefit from, but this obviously translates across the board to more important choices and decisions.

We have been conditioned since birth

I am very grateful to my partner, Mary, who introduced me to Dr Maria Montessori's book *The Absorbent Mind* a few years ago. Mary was studying to become a Montessori teacher, and took me to a conference in London to learn more about how the brain of a child develops. Prior to this, I had already published a book which went into the workings of the subconscious and conscious mind, but I was unaware of the Italian physician and educator Maria Montessori who pioneered research in this area way back in the 1920s and 1930s. I was fascinated with the concepts in *The Absorbent Mind*, and it reaffirmed the importance of nurturing a child's subconscious mind with love, compassion, mindfulness, abundance and confidence from an early age. Dr Montessori wrote:

> Others, after having studied children carefully, have come to the conclusion that the first two years are the most important of life. Education during this period must be intended as a help to the development of the psychic powers inherent in the human individual.

While many were raised with enlightened parents who deliberately worked to enhance their children's confidence and nurtured them with non-shaming feedback, a great many people were conditioned with quite the opposite. If you do not believe me, pay attention to some of the interactions you witness between young children and their parents/carers in public places.

We were conditioned from the moment of birth. Our subconscious mind was wide open to suggestion, and our parents, family of origin and environment played a huge role in shaping our brains. Like a sponge, we absorbed the thoughts, feelings, emotions and sensations of those closely associated to us. We therefore internalized their thoughts, feelings, emotions and sensations, which left an imprint on us. We were given a programme, which became a subconscious programme, because we could not remember every exact moment or feeling we experienced. An unhelpful comment by a great uncle regarding your physical features may still be haunting you today. A crass comment on your potential as a child may have left a deep emotional imprint in your brain and body, which may be stifling your potential to thrive in some way. The point is, we cannot possibly consciously remember every thought, feeling and emotion we absorbed at this tender age, but the deeper layers of our mind do. The human body certainly remembers everything, and as we depend on our bodies to take action and to get things moving in our lives, you will see how powerful such early subconscious programming is. We will cover how to overwrite and create our own conditioning in the final two chapters.

'It runs in the family'

Have your parents or members of your family of origin ever said to you that your behaviour or the behaviour of another family member 'runs in the family'? Or told you 'you're a chip off the old block'? They are probably right! Very often, subconscious patterns of behaviour trickle down through generations. Some of the time, such patterns of behaviours may skip a generation or two, but if we trace back and investigate our family of origin, we will notice similar patterns of behaviour. This is why almost every person I have met recovering from addictive or co-dependent behaviour will realize that addiction was a generational problem. While we are all unique individuals, there is an unconscious field of energy (emotions, sensations, thoughts, perceptions of reality) which pass down the generations going back hundreds of years. Many of our attitudes towards work, business, education, politics and social issues have been unconsciously shaped for us. Our parents may have differing views from ourselves, but we may trace an uncle or aunt or a grandparent who had similar views to ourselves regarding various business, social and political issues. Human beings are highly complicated, and there is certainly a grey area regarding our early conditioning, but make no mistake, our family of origin has programmed us. There was no other way we could have learned to eat, talk, walk, read and write, let alone absorbed the tens of thousands of conversations we were exposed to in the first three years of our lives. The good news is that we do not have to play out old family scripts. We can individuate and become our true selves, and shape our brains in a way which resonates with our true desires.

The emotional brain is faster than your thinking brain

One of the examples I give in my lectures and seminars regarding the emotional brain being faster than your thinking brain is to imagine for a moment approaching physical danger. You are walking down a busy high street and all of a sudden three lions appear from nowhere and begin making their way towards you. Some of the crowd in the high street begin screaming and running away, while others freeze in terror. In this very moment, your limbic system, particularly the amygdala and your brainstem, will kick in. Your fight, flight, freeze and faint responses will take over your behaviour. Whichever survival reaction is strongest will determine whether you run away, fight back, freeze or faint. In other words, when real perceived danger is present your body will take over. There is no time to ponder on what to do when three hungry lions are running towards you. You will act swiftly without thinking. The reason the emotional brain has this supreme control during perceived threats is because it is truly ancient. The brainstem is over 300 million years old. The limbic system (your emotional brain) is over 100 million years old. Conversely, the prefrontal cortex, which is an instrument for thinking and reason, is 4 million years old. The emotional brain, 'the old guard', has had hundreds of millions of years to establish itself in the body, throughout the changes in evolution.

When we attempt to change our life by just rationalizing and thinking, we are wasting our time. The only way to get our emotional brain and body to cooperate with us is to speak the language it understands, which is *emotion*.

Entrenched limiting beliefs

Ingrained limiting beliefs are a result of being in a firmly established hypnotic trance. Essentially, for many of us with entrenched limiting beliefs, we have adopted disempowering ideas about ourselves and the world, and we are dominated by them. Even after my sixth book, *The Kindness Habit*, had been published in 2016, which I co-authored with Dr Barbara Mariposa and had a foreword written by the late John Bradshaw, I noticed my emotions suggesting that I was wasting my time writing books. Where did these subtle, subliminal feelings come from? Intellectually speaking, I could not deny that I was adding value to society, but layers of unresolved shame and fear still pestered me. I remember receiving a sincere email from a reader regarding the value she received from one of my earlier books, and out of nowhere I had thoughts like 'She's just being nice' and 'My work is still not good enough.'

We can have limiting beliefs about all sorts of things in our lives. The key thing to remember is that an emotion always underlies a belief. If you catch yourself believing you cannot progress in your recovery or any other area of your life, ask yourself what the feeling is behind this belief. There you will find what is holding you back from progressing.

The critical inner voice

Almost all of us have a critical inner voice, often referred to as the critical inner parent or 'the monkey on your shoulder'. It often generates fear, anxiety and self-doubt. I have come to realize that the critical inner voice is our subconscious programming. It especially becomes louder when we try to change our lives for the better. If we wish to get involved in a healthy romantic relationship but have a track record of disappointing romantic relationships, rest assured that the critical inner voice will remind you why you will probably fail. If you try to set up a successful business or attempt to spread your wings and really go for your dream career, the critical inner voice will be telling you otherwise. I refer to this mental noise as a voice because there are hundreds of monologues and silent conversations operating in our minds. The critical inner voice is a manifestation of our subconscious thoughts and feelings. The next time you find yourself talking yourself out of what could be a good idea, write down in your notebook what your critical inner voice is suggesting and discuss it with a person who is consciously working on improving their lives. The critical inner voice needs to be challenged, and a good listening ear from a sympathetic person or recovery partner will help you to transcend your disempowering feelings.

Unconsciously seeking chaos

Many shame-based people will find ways to mask their traumatic memories and feelings by unconsciously recreating chaotic lifestyles which reflect their unpredictable childhood experiences. Other extreme behaviours may manifest in sitting on the sidelines of life. They watch others fully engaged in life and are utterly baffled by their own lack of ability to do the same. Black-and-white thinking clouds their ability to look deeper into the complexities of life. In some cases, extreme vagueness dominates their life.

While adrenaline certainly serves an important purpose primarily to protect a person from potential physical threats, emotionally wounded and highly addictive personalities will use adrenaline in the same way that a drug addict will abuse opioids or a compulsive debtor will max out three credit cards.

With hindsight, I realize that I myself used adrenaline to alter the way I felt. For example, I could easily numb out at school by creating conflict with school teachers and my fellow students. I used to verbally antagonize students who were physically stronger than me to provoke a reaction and therefore create an adrenaline rush, even if it cost me a black eye. In my first ten years of total abstinence, I still found myself creating adrenaline rushes but on a much smaller scale. I found ways to cram in as many activities as possible just before I was due to attend an important appointment, resulting in me being late and thereby provoking a jolt of adrenaline. I used to do this before I travelled to a different country. I would leave it to the very last minute to make my way to the airport and put myself through an emotional cocktail of excitement, anticipation and adrenaline. It is only when I hit another rock bottom 11 years into my recovery and got honest about my adrenaline addiction that I gained enough self-awareness to change my behaviour.

Being charged with adrenaline might help to numb emotional pain in the short to medium term. However, it will eventually take its toll on the human body. Furthermore, it is not natural to go through life without allowing ourselves to feel our emotions.

Conscious and subconscious levels of awareness

There are many levels of self-awareness, but for now let us focus on two primary levels of awareness: the conscious and subconscious. For example, when you constantly tell yourself (at an emotional level) that you are not capable of being in a loving, romantic, long-term relationship because you have a track record of being in dysfunctional romantic relationships, your subconscious level of awareness hears this: *I am going to deny myself being in a loving, romantic, long-term relationship.* When you tell yourself over and over again that you cannot improve your life because of your current circumstances, your subconscious awareness hears this: *I am going to deny myself an opportunity to change my current circumstances.* If you continue to rewire your brain, fuelled with emotion, your body will mirror such conditioning through your behaviour. Your body cannot reject an emotion for every feeling will leave an imprint.

In ancient Greece and during the Roman Empire, the word 'heart' meant the subconscious mind. The ancient saying 'As a man thinketh in his heart, so is he' (Proverbs 23:7) is a wise one. Some of our more enlightened ancestors intuitively realized that there were two primary levels of awareness. The conscious mind might be attempting to take a particular course of action, whereas the subconscious mind, 'the heart', could have entirely different plans. In his book *As a Man Thinketh*, James Allen has written: 'We think in secret and it comes to pass, environment is but a looking glass.' Notice how Allen emphasized thinking in secret, meaning at a subconscious level and undetectable to the conscious mind. Thus, our results are but the looking glass (a mirror) of our subconscious programming.

Most of us feel stuck in our lives because we have been programmed to behave in such a way. This is why talking with others in recovery about their own challenges of changing their behaviour is so helpful, because such a conversation can help to access buried memories and emotions.

2

Reducing the feelings of unworthiness

Unlike guilt, which is the feeling of doing something wrong shame is the feeling of being something wrong.

Marilyn J. Sorensen

Unfortunately, many people feel utterly flawed at the core of their being. For example, a shame-based person might feel like a failure if they make a mistake at work, home or in a social gathering. Making an error to a shame-based person will cause burning embarrassment, self-pity, misplaced guilt and a feeling of unworthiness. The reaction to making a human mistake is way out of proportion to the error made. They might even rage because the illusion of perfection has once again been challenged. By contrast, a person with a healthy sense of self will acknowledge when an error has been made but will not automatically feel fatally flawed. I used to feel like I was a mistake until I got into recovery and started the process of personal and spiritual growth. We will cover solutions to feeling unworthy at the end of this chapter.

Shameless behaviour is driven by 'all or nothing' thinking

Shame-based people tend to act shamelessly and have little regard for their own human limitations. Their relationships with others are often shallow. They use people for their own gain and discard them when they are no longer useful. In many respects, I used to be a shameless person. While in active drug and alcohol addiction, I used people for my own self-seeking motives. People were either useful or they were not – my thinking was very black and white – 'all or nothing'. I found it hard to sustain relationships and was baffled when people turned on me. Until I sobered up, I could not truly see how I was treating myself and others. It was very hard looking at my shortcomings and shameless behaviour when I first took a fearless and thorough inventory for the first time in my first year in recovery. I had to feel and own my shame for the first time without a mind- and mood-altering substance to numb the discomfort. Feeling my shame and emotional pain brought me humility and some degree of clarity. Seeing clearly how I used to behave has helped me to be much more empathetic and compassionate towards myself and others. We need to be able to empathize with others if we are going to respect our own human limitations and not behave in shameless ways.

If I draw upon my own experience, and that of the many people I have observed over the years, it is not possible to be true to our own values and demonstrate courage if we still feel fatally flawed and unlovable. A shame-based, emotionally wounded person will have to work very hard to bury the chronic shame they carry inside. This is incredibly tiring and uses up energy which could otherwise be channelled into more productive outlets. Until a shame-based person gets into recovery, they have no choice but to create a false self. What other option do they have? Creating a false self, and inauthentic character traits, is a matter of survival.

We cannot be empathetic towards others and avoid shameless behaviour if we are unable to connect with our true selves. To connect with our true selves takes a lot of commitment, patience and willingness. Adult children of narcissists, adult children of alcoholics and drug addicts, and adult children who grew up in highly dysfunctional families, tend to be chronically shame-based people, and often identify with a false self, when they start their recovery process. I highly recommend reading John Bradshaw's classic book, *Healing the Shame That Binds You*. Bradshaw was a pioneer of shame-based, deep feeling work, and inner-child recovery. In his book, Bradshaw goes into great detail how toxic shame causes us to behave in dysfunctional ways such as addictive behaviours and co-dependency. He outlines practical solutions and includes his personal experience of healing from toxic shame.

Self-abandoning behaviour

Shame-based people who were betrayed and abandoned in childhood and adolescence often abandon themselves. They may constantly have sex with strangers, rather than getting to know a person and have some sort of fulfilling emotional connection. They may sabotage their efforts to succeed in the material world. They may persist in trying to befriend people who are not really interested in them. Self-abandoning behaviour is essentially recreating abandonment and betrayal in our adult life. For example, I used to casually date women who were emotionally unavailable and just wanted sex. While that may have been convenient at first, after a while this pattern of behaviour became deeply unsatisfactory at an emotional and spiritual level. This was self-abandoning behaviour.

The difficulty in overcoming self-abandonment is that it is very often unconscious behaviour. Some of us are so deeply ingrained in our survival traits, and swamped in self-delusion, that we cannot see when we are neglecting ourselves. It is extremely difficult to heal from self-abandoning behaviour without help. We need non-shaming people to mirror back to us our disempowering behaviour. I needed people in my support group to hold a space for me to make mistakes, learn from them, and change my behaviour. I needed patient and loving people who were willing to reflect back my thoughts and feelings.

Wanting to be saved by someone

When a young child does not have her emotional needs met within the first two to three years she will develop a false self to survive. Her thinking will most likely be 'all or nothing'. As the emotionally wounded child grows up, she creates a fantasy that one day new parental figures will save her and give her the emotional nourishment she so desperately needs. Think how many people are yearning for a 'father figure' or a 'mother figure', hoping to be validated. The truth is that no one can save us in adulthood. To be a mature adult is to respect death and be aware that we must take care of ourselves, with the assistance of our fellow human beings. We will all die one day, and no human being can prevent this from happening. When we fully accept our mortality (at a human level), our spiritual practice can expand and deepen.

While there is a part of emotionally undeveloped people which yearns to be 'taken care of', emotionally intelligent adults accept that they are responsible for their own lives. They create their own reality, consciously or unconsciously, moment to moment. They accept that they need help from others but are not too dependent on anyone (unless they are physically disabled, mentally impaired or seriously ill). They have developed an internal resource of resilience, self-awareness and humility.

Until I learned to re-parent myself in adulthood, I was still unconsciously wishing that someone or something would 'save me' or 'rescue me' from my deep emotional wounds and woes, which was a manifestation of an arrested emotional development (untreated drug addicts, alcoholics and co-dependents all have an arrested emotional development, before they do some serious work on their emotional and spiritual development). While I was still secretly wishing to be saved by a powerful institution or an influential person in my previous career, I was still operating from a place of neediness and consequently I was easily manipulated. My unhealed wounds and entrenched grief were the driving force behind this behaviour. Today I have compassion for my adolescent self and for the young adult who was trying to make sense of life without the aid of alcohol and drugs.

Feeling ashamed about career and creative stagnation

Career stagnation can cause us to feel ashamed about our lives. It can dent our self-belief and affect our personal relationships. It is one thing to feel stuck in a job – it is another thing to feel ashamed as a person in a stagnating and unfulfilling career. A person may have finished his training at law school and find that he loathes the mundane nature of much of his day-to-day work in his career of choice. He feels ashamed to admit this to his family and friends.

In my previous music career, I knew of several high-profile DJs and producers who felt lost, despite being established and financially stable. They had lost their passion and enthusiasm for their work but, being in their fifties, felt that it was too late to retrain in a different field. The shame and embarrassment of walking away from their field was causing them to self-sabotage in all sorts of ways.

Creative artistic stagnation is often caused by fear and shame. It is hard to access a creative inner spark if we are holding on to chronic shame. In order to create, we have to have to address our fears whenever they arise so that we can keep a clear channel open to receive inspiration. This is why I suggest group meditation to people who have artistic stagnation. We will be re-energized and inspired by accessing moments of stillness. Travelling is another wonderful way to rejuvenate the human spirit and form new ideas. If it is not possible to travel abroad, there are plenty of awe-inspiring locations in every country on earth. The key thing is to try to experience something new – travel to a new location, meet new people, listen to a new album or watch an excellent new film. Creative inspiration has to be nurtured through new experiences. Romance and making love can enhance creativity. Similarly, sexual energy (the desire for sex and sexual pleasure) used constructively can be channelled into creative works.

Shame attacks in a toxic working environment

According to the people I have worked with over the years, one of the biggest triggers is the workplace. Very often, a workplace is a breeding ground for pathological competitiveness, resentment, jealousy and apathy. Many employees are considered numbers on a spreadsheet. Staff welfare all too often takes a backseat in many organizations. While some working environments nurture fulfilment, wellbeing and wellness in staff, many companies are a painful part of people's lives. This is often a result of most people feeling apathy and resentment towards their jobs. When people feel trapped in a hostile working environment, rest assured that a scapegoat will be created, especially in an office. Blame and 'passing the buck' are a given in such working environments. A bullying culture can easily become prevalent, and perpetrators and victims will appear. Very often, this behaviour trickles down from the very top of an organization.

For people healing from trauma, frozen grief and addictions, working in a hostile, unfriendly environment can trigger all sorts of problems. The fact is, some employers and employees are so unaware of their own lack of personal boundaries and sensitivity toward others that they can have a devastating ripple effect in a business. Controlling and rescuing others becomes a way to try to resolve wounds from the past. Unconsciously, many people attract working environments which reflect their upbringing, due to their unconscious patterns of behaviour. They attract working environments which reflect their subconscious beliefs, ideas and vibrational frequency. Some people have a moment of clarity and realize that they have been doing this, and so they take a step back and begin to work on their own emotional and spiritual recovery. However, most people will go through their entire working life neglecting their own wellness and settling for disempowering working environments.

The only way through this is to reach out and be willing to receive help from people who have more experience than us, professionally speaking. We will need a lot of support and a new trajectory. The fact is no one is forced to work in a particular job or in an industry. We can make a decision to change course, regardless of age, gender, race or religion. Fear and anxiety might very well appear while making a course correction, but we can ride out these temporary emotional fluctuations as we make our plans to create a meaningful and fulfilling career.

Misplaced guilt

Guilt is imperative if we are to create and sustain a decent code of ethics and a sound moral compass. Guilt can help us to listen to our conscience, enhance empathy, and therefore have fulfilling relationships. Without guilt, we would live in an extremely dark world. However, misplaced guilt often triggers us to be over-apologetic and people-please. Many people repeat the word 'sorry' without needing to, while still others feel guilty for their very own existence. Emotionally wounded, shame-based people often feel that they are constantly 'getting in the way'. This stems from a sense of feeling unlovable. To ask for one's own needs to be met often results in a feeling of guilt. I call this misplaced guilt. Similarly, a person may feel guilty even if they have been abused or harmed by others. Misplaced guilt or excessive guilt stifles people's chances to live happily and peacefully.

Life can be messy

Have you heard the saying by the actor Lily Tomlin, 'The road to success is always under construction'? I like this concept. My spiritual journey has certainly been messy and uncomfortable at times. I had several emotional breakdowns before experiencing an emotional breakthrough. In essence, layers of deep denial and negative thought-patterns had to be unravelled and replaced with new and greater self-awareness.

The nature of life is change and movement, and so people and things are always going to evolve, including me. This is bound to create some degree of disruption. The key thing in life is to continue to seek to progress in our own unique way. Stagnation and complacency are abhorrent to nature. If we are to live in harmony with life, we are required to evolve, and by doing so we will experience a certain level of emotional discomfort.

My friend Kelly McNelis, founder of Women For One, has written an excellent book on life being messy. In *Your Messy Brilliance*, Kelly shares her experience, regarding coming through incredible personal challenges and learning to let go of perfectionism. Although her book is written for women, her approach to emotional and spiritual recovery is universal. Kelly's courage is felt throughout her talks and articles. She writes:

> Many of us are walking around in a state of self-delusion and guardedness, regardless of whether or not we have experienced trauma in early life. In a twisted way, this is part of the human condition. We internalize the tragedy and shame of our experiences to such an extent that we end up locking ourselves behind iron fortresses. In our need to keep ourselves from being hurt, we deny the very parts

of our being that most need our unconditional love and acceptance.

Kelly outlines the following major subjects in her book: curiosity, awareness, acceptance, intuition, choice, manifestation and the infinite roadmap.

Chronic body shame

To be insecure makes us human and is a natural process of life. While going through puberty, it would be abnormal not to compare our bodies with those around us and at times want to look different. However, if we have reached adulthood and are still highly insecure about our bodies, we may need to do some more work on ourselves to diminish our self-loathing. Chronic body shame has caused immense suffering and embarrassment for people all over the world. Women often feel insecure after giving birth if they are unable to lose weight or have been left with stretch marks around their bellies. Many young men feel insecure for not having a compelling, athletic body. Ageing can trigger shame: wrinkles, stretch marks, saggy skin, baldness or hair growth. Young people in particular are constantly bombarded by images of the 'perfect' body on popular social media platforms. Social media apps have heightened the obsession with a 'flawless appearance'.

Certainly, since the 1980s the cult of global celebrity has certainly played its part in creating unattainable images and expectations in fans' minds. The 1950s to the 1980s produced 'godlike' movie and pop stars. Although both pop and movie stars do not shine as brightly in the twenty-first century as they once did in the twentieth century, star power is still a compelling force in shaping cultural norms. However, celebrities are often at the mercy of marketing forces and campaigns. Social media influencers are often pressured to comply to corporate pressure, even though they are deemed to be trendsetters themselves.

There is nothing wrong with wanting to change our physical appearance. It can help to enhance self-esteem and boost self-confidence. The problem arises when our physical appearance becomes all-consuming and we neglect to take care of our inner world – our spiritual and emotional life.

Puberty for almost all children can be very unsettling. I hated it when my body started to change. I was unable to talk about these changes during my childhood and early adolescence. It was only in adulthood that I could talk to other men about how utterly difficult it was. For instance, I started dating girls my age by the time I was 12 or 13 and therefore attracted girls of my age and slightly older who were also sexually active. Many of my friends at school did not start dating girls until they were 15. Within a space of 12 months, I started to grow hair on my body, which was baffling. I did not talk to anyone at the time, although I had learned about the absolute basics of puberty at school. I later found out that some of my friends at the time were embarrassed not to have any hair on their body in their early teens. At one point, I had a lot of spots and felt very self-conscious. I remember the very first time a teacher told me to have a shower with my school friends, after a swimming class. I cannot explain the shame and embarrassment I felt leading up to that shower. I was terrified that I would be mocked for having a smaller penis than my classmates. Alcohol and cannabis certainly helped to soothe my fear and anxiety back then.

I remember hearing a man over 15 years sober at a rehab share how he had a dreadful time during puberty. He, too, felt as though he had the 'oddest' body as a boy and was convinced that he had the smallest penis in the world. Like me, he found refuge in alcohol. I have listened to many women in recovery from drug/alcohol addiction and co-dependency who were raised in a dysfunctional family and who were consumed with fear regarding the size of their breasts.

Some of them were embarrassed to have had large breasts as young teenage girls, while others felt terribly insecure as a result of having small breasts.

Children and young adolescents are highly intuitive and my classmates were brutal. If they spotted a sensitive side in a friend, vitriol and mockery would soon follow. A reasonably emotionally grounded adolescent will be able to grow through puberty and come through young adulthood without carrying too many emotional scars. However, many shame-based people are carrying unaddressed emotional wounds well into middle age. In my case, I had to revisit the shame of puberty and make peace with my past shame and embarrassment.

Four months after I stopped drinking alcohol I received a request to DJ in Thailand. It was my second trip to Thailand, having spent the previous year drinking and taking drugs while on a highly dysfunctional DJ tour. However, when I returned to Thailand for the first time during my recovery, I felt incredibly embarrassed to swim with my friends. My promoter at the time lived in Thailand and looked after an opulent mansion which had a large swimming pool right next to the sea. I never felt comfortable swimming with her unless it was dark outside. She was aware of my being a few months clean and, thankfully for me, was non-shaming.

A similar incident happened the following year when I attended a week's convention for recovering addicts in Marbella. I was among people who had taken me under their wing and yet I was unable to swim in the hotel swimming pool due to feeling utterly ashamed by my body. A woman, ten years my senior, from my support group in north London, frankly asked me why I had avoided the swimming pool all week. She knew what was going on with me because we had listened to each other share shameful and harrowing memories at our local support group. She pointed out that most of our group felt triggered because it was the first time in years that many of us had been on holiday while stone-cold sober. We had to feel the emotions we masked during puberty, which for many of us felt like being utterly exposed. Thankfully, I have been able to work through my body shame, as a result of talking about it. Common thoughts and feelings regarding body shame are:

- I'm ugly.
- I'm disgusting.
- I'm just full of fat and flab.
- I'll never be attractive.
- I'm just not attractive.
- I feel and look like shit.
- Why can't I look like X?
- I never look good in the mirror.
- My wrinkles make me look unattractive.
- I'm ashamed of my body.
- If only my skin wasn't so pale.
- If only my skin wasn't so dark.
- I hate how my teeth look.
- I'm covered in moles and freckles.

A distorted view of one's physical appearance can trigger harmful addictive behaviours, which can lead to severe eating disorders (particularly bulimia and anorexia). Many recovering alcoholics, co-dependents and drug addicts from my support groups have battled with eating disorders due to loathing what they see in the mirror.

According to Dr Keon West, of Goldsmiths, University of London, naturism has a positive psychological effect on people who loathe the appearance of their bodies. People with a low regard for their physical appearance can improve their self-esteem by spending time with people, on a non-intimate basis, while *completely naked*. The idea is for highly self-conscious people to spend time with confident non-shaming naked people and join them in collective activities such as sunbathing and

23

walking together in nature. According to Dr West's studies and the Channel 4 documentary *Naked Beach* which he features in, highly self-conscious people reported an improvement in their physical self-image and a boost to their self-esteem. One of the suggestions made to those struggling to like their bodies was to stand in the mirror naked for 20 minutes every evening for a week. By looking at oneself in the mirror, shame attacks are reduced. The first night was painfully awkward but, by the end of the week, those participating in the study felt less ashamed of their bodies.

While chronic body-shame is a horrible thing to live with, especially if one is publicly shamed on the internet, in some cases dissatisfaction can be a catalyst for people to take appropriate action. Like most things in life, there is seldom a black-and-white, all–or–nothing solution. Addressing body-shame is very personal and with an open mind and a willingness to heal the shame we carry inside of us, we can find an appropriate way which works for us.

Coming to terms with our shame

The more we try to disassociate from our shame, relying solely on our own reasoning and will power in an attempt to get some emotional relief, the stronger the hold shame has over us. Our shame-based behaviour will find ways to reveal itself if we remain in denial about our pain. Shame can be very subtle and often operates at a subconscious level of awareness. However, when we accept we are carrying unresolved shame, we can heal and make peace with ourselves.

With respect to my own shame, I can still feel like hiding from life. I have found that listening to people talking about their shame has helped me to identify my own shame-based triggers and given me the courage to be authentic. I especially need to be honest with myself, as a result of writing books on personal growth, mindfulness and recovery. When I started facilitating self-referral and corporate seminars in my mid-twenties, I was still quite brash. However, life has humbled me some more, and I am much more in tune with my own feelings.

We can feel ashamed for all sorts of reasons:

- We have never been able to sustain a committed romantic relationship.
- We have never been in a committed loving, erotic relationship.
- We are not earning enough money to live financially prosperously.
- We do not have the confidence to meet new people in social gatherings. Therefore, we hide from social engagements.
- We are afraid to travel the world and experience new cultures. We are afraid something bad might happen to us if we leave the 'safety' of our own country.
- We do not have meaningful friendships.
- We dislike or are embarrassed by our physical appearance.
- We have not realized many of our dreams and desires. We may feel like a failure.
- We have made a lot of mistakes as a parent or carer to our offspring.
- We have made mistakes which we cannot change, and this still disturbs our peace of mind.
- We have long-term ill health.

Proven tools to address feelings of unworthiness

Here are some proven tools to help you to reduce feelings of chronic shame and unworthiness. They have worked for me, my friends and clients as well as scores of other people in recovery. I have personally mentored people through the process outlined below and it works. These proven tools to address feelings of unworthiness will bring good results, but the process of healing shame-based emotions takes time. We can speed up manifesting desires, once we have addressed our shame. Until then, our frozen shame and self-contempt will keep us stuck. In other words, we have to address our feelings of unworthiness before we can thrive in life.

- Join a weekly support group. This can be a face-to-face support group or a conference call/online group. We cannot overcome feelings of unworthiness by ourselves.
- *Ask* a non-shaming, compassionate and experienced mentor to assist you to work through your unconscious and subconscious shame-based emotions. You can *attract* such a mentor by deciding to. This can be a good therapist or mentor who has worked through their own shame-based emotions. For example, in a Twelve Step community (a fellowship that uses the Twelve Step programme of recovery from addiction as pioneered by Alcoholics Anonymous), a member will typically have a 'sponsor', meaning a mentor to guide them through the process of recovery.
- Take up mindfulness as a practice. A local mindfulness meditation group can certainly help a great deal. There are plenty of guided meditations available online and to purchase. I have created several guided scripted meditations in this book in later chapters.
- Develop the habit of sharing your emotional state with non-shaming people who are working on their own recovery from unworthiness and shame. Make sure you trust and respect them, and they trust and respect you. It might take some time to attract such people, but your willingness and desire to meet them will bring them to you.
- Look into your eyes in the mirror at least once a day for 30 seconds or longer. Gradually, negative emotions about yourself will melt away. Do this for a month and report back to your mentor and/or support group.

- Invest in a journal and make a note of your current feelings, and discuss them with your mentor. You will get some relief by writing down your feelings, but you will heal by exposing your emotions with another human being. You will probably meet with embarrassment while sharing your findings, but remember that this is part of the healing process. This will help you to process and discard such emotions. Below is an example of my journal:

11 July 2016
I was in a lot of emotional pain today, and I felt angry because I did not reach financial targets this month. I need to change my approach and ask for some guidance. I am frustrated.

2 May 2016
I dissociated on Saturday evening by binge-watching a documentary series on Netflix to numb my grief and pain. I was feeling numb and alone.

3 May 2016
I wept for an hour before attending a recovery group. I wept again on Sunday night. I believe this was linked to my frozen grief work.

8 October 2017
I'm feeling embarrassed and ashamed again about the way my body looks. This shame vanished last year while I was doing my major frozen grief work, but it's reared its ugly head again. I have had a shame attack and feel conscious about the way I look. I know this feeling will pass, and so I've just got to feel it until it passes.

9 October 2017
I'm feeling much better today. I'm feeling grateful for my life and much more optimistic about my prospects. I received a call from an old friend, which cheered me up.

3

The power of gentleness and vulnerability

> When we were children, we used to think that when we
> were grown-up we would no longer be vulnerable. But to
> grow up is to accept vulnerability ... To be alive is to be
> vulnerable.
>
> *Madeleine L'Engle*

As a person recovering from multiple addictive behaviours, I
have come to see how important practising super self-care has
been in my life. Practising radical self-care has helped me to
make peace with myself, enhanced my humanness and created
long-lasting friendships. For those of us who have learned to
live with a mental illness (or being dual-diagnosis), it serves
us well to practise self-love. Our emotional and spiritual life
ultimately depends on a willingness to treat ourselves with the
utmost respect. I benefit greatly by being gentle with myself and
being able to bring humour into everyday living. Benevolence,
laughter and self-compassion keeps me sober, playful and
energized, whereas self-neglect keeps me compulsively seeking
external validation and trapped in survival mode.

Although I came into recovery to address my drug and alcohol
addictions, I subsequently experienced further rock bottoms
regarding my process addictions and had to embark upon a
process of stripping away my false self. The biggest disruptor was
coming to terms with major frozen grief and the realization that
I needed to proceed with deep-feeling grief work. I had been 11
years without drinking alcohol and taking drugs; I had previously thought that I had addressed my major emotional pain by

engaging with a programme regarding love addiction and love avoidance in my early twenties, but I was soon to discover that there was another thick layer of grief to process. I also identify as a compulsive hider (many compulsive under-earners identify with compulsive hiding) – someone who finds it impossible to remain visible in all areas of life. It is not possible to be successful in this world without being consistently, authentically visible. To be a successful school teacher, banker, athlete, bar tender or a pop star requires sustained visibility. In my view, my compulsive hiding is linked with my emotional triggers, frozen grief and trauma. A person must be exposed and therefore vulnerable in order to practise visibility.

Gentleness serves us well

Being gentle with ourselves in an organic way allows us to find refuge and access serenity. Gentleness helps us to learn from our mistakes without being hard on ourselves. We can learn from making a mistake without attacking ourselves. For example, how does it serve us to tell ourselves to 'man up' if we are dying from alcoholism or an eating disorder? How does it serve us to refer to ourselves as 'stupid' for not being able to 'cure' ourselves of depression or drug addiction? Vitriol directed inwards only makes matters worse. The more we continue to tell ourselves that we are stupid for making mistakes, the more we are inclined to believe all sorts of cruel things about ourselves. We thereby diminish ourselves.

Many of us have been undermining ourselves for decades without realizing it. We have neglected to take care of our basic human needs and wants such as having loving relationships, genuine friendships and a healthy vibrant lifestyle. We have starved ourselves of love and compassion. We have denied ourselves new experiences, as a result of being rigid and obsessed with controlling people and outcomes. Many of us have pretended for years that we have no desire for creative or intellectually stimulating hobbies and projects. Some of us have stayed in well-paid jobs which we utterly loathed. Many of us have been subject to all sorts of severe abuse and neglect. We even punished ourselves for the abuse we received. However, we can learn to direct gentleness inwards and feel the benefits of tenderness and benevolence.

Gentleness accepts the truth but approaches it with kindness

While it might have been true that, during my active alcoholism and drug addiction, I was causing damage to myself and others, it was a gentle support group and fellowship that helped me to heal. My first recovery mentor was a softly spoken and warm-hearted American/British musician. He could empathize with my passion for playing music and battling with drug addiction at a young age. He was exactly what I needed because I was mentally, emotionally, spiritually, physically and financially destitute. Since then I have had various mentors with differing temperaments. Two years later I got in touch with my anger for the first time without using alcohol and illegal drugs, and so I was drawn to very angry people. However, after a few years, I realized that I had to go deeper than my anger and get in touch my immense sadness, loneliness, loss and arrested grief.

We can be honest with ourselves without being harsh and unkind. For instance, we might acknowledge that we have to address yet 'another' addictive behaviour. One day we might look in the mirror and acknowledge that we need to lose some weight or maybe gain some. We might realize that our spending habits are causing us severe stress and financial difficulties. We might have a moment of clarity and realize that we cannot cure a loved one from drug and alcohol addiction. Rather than harshly condemning ourselves, we can accept life *as it is* and ask for help.

Gentleness enhances meditation

Meditation is a powerful practice which can help us to heal our emotional pain. To observe our thoughts and feelings requires willingness and gentleness. We cannot be rigid and harsh on ourselves and hope to feel serene. We have to be willing to go easy on ourselves. The only way to be present and gain the benefits of mindfulness is to love ourselves unconditionally. This is a gradual process. All of us can experience self-doubt. However, some of us are utterly consumed with self-doubt, which is often a manifestation of chronic shame, abandonment and unaddressed grief. The important thing to remember is to be gentle on ourselves when self-doubt manifests in our minds. It is an opportunity to be vulnerable with our support network and process our feelings without numbing out. We can talk, trust and feel. If we have a passing thought which suggests that we are 'pathetic' or 'ugly', we can witness the thought and have compassion for ourselves. If we begin to clench our jaws or perspiration runs down our foreheads, as a result of being triggered by a traumatic memory, we can soothe ourselves by taking a deep breath. We can affirm that we are safe and capable of practising super self-care. For those of us who believe in a higher power, we can say a prayer after taking several deep slow breaths.

When a group of people come together to meditate, there tends to be a collective calm. The collective consciousness is often soothing or tranquil. People tend to loosen up and feel relaxed. Their stress levels have reduced, and they therefore approach others with affection and consideration. Whether an emotionally wounded person is practising mindfulness, yoga, transcendental meditation, box breathing or any other meditation, a gentle approach is required to fully feel the benefits of meditation.

There is power in being vulnerable

Every time I call a friend and take a risk in sharing how I am truly feeling, I expand my self-awareness. There is power in being vulnerable. First, it is a process of surrendering to the present moment. Second, I get a sense of relief by sharing my emotions with a non-shaming friend. Third, I feel more connected to my fellow human beings. I consequently feel part of a pack. If I subsequently need to weep as a result of talking about my emotions, then I can heal some more. If I feel lighter and cheerful as a result of being vulnerable with a friend, then I gladly accept this too.

I see the power of vulnerability every time I attend a support group and hear men and women share their experience, strength and hope. When a man breaks down in a Twelve Step meeting and has got in touch with his frozen grief, he has started the process of profound deep healing. I, too, benefit as a result of listening to his suffering because it helps me to connect with my own suffering. Whenever a person attends therapy or a support group, they are practising vulnerability. Every time I share my joy or sadness with my support group, I am coming out of hiding ('coming out of the cave') and developing courage. I can still emotionally connect with a person who is two days dry from alcohol addiction because I can relate to his or her vulnerability; it helps me to reflect.

Considering the appropriate time to be vulnerable is essential. It might not be appropriate to disclose sensitive information to a person who is emotionally unavailable. This is often a process of trial and error until we have established a safe support network.

There is no doubt that vulnerability is becoming less 'shameful' in today's society. Social media is brimming with people living with a mental illness who are sharing their stories of hope. The 'Me Too' movement is another example of both men and women coming out of hiding and disclosing their pain and frozen grief. There is nothing shameful about accepting help. It takes courage to be open to receive assistance.

Visibility means being exposed

What do you feel when the word 'exposed' comes to mind? Do you feel afraid and anxious? One of the biggest stumbling blocks I had regarding my personal and professional goals was the fear of being visible and exposed. Sustaining visibility without help was emotionally taxing. The problem was, I had no idea that I was afraid of visibility. For example, I sabotaged a lot of opportunities in my previous music career due to feeling exposed. To be exposed and visible meant being open to being criticized, and, for a shame/fear-based, emotionally wounded person, that was too risky. When I felt my feelings for the first time as an adult, I had to gradually learn to process my emotions. This was a process of trial and error. For example, with regard to my creative projects I could sustain visibility for short spells, but then I would retreat and go back into hiding. I was easily triggered. I have come to realize that a human being can be addicted to hiding – hiding from opportunities to prosper, hiding from being visible, and hiding from life.

If we are going to be of maximum service to our fellow human beings in our own unique way, this will require a willingness to be exposed. It means that our fellow co-workers, employers and employees will see our weaknesses as well as our strengths. Some will criticize us and maybe gossip about us. We will be triggered at times. We may feel angry and frustrated, but the pros so often outweigh the cons. To be ourselves and to be visible means that we are far more likely to attract the kind of people we wish to associate with. We are far more likely to succeed in this world if we are prepared to show up and take risks. All areas of my life improved when I became authentically visible. My challenge today is to sustain my authentic visibility, one day at a time.

It is by no means easy, and at times the fear of visibility can be unsettling. To be visible is truly *living*.

Courage is a practice

To be gentle with ourselves requires a willingness to be exposed and perhaps be hurt. As I have already suggested, there is nothing weak or 'cowardly' about gentleness, especially when we are relearning to live in this world by minimizing our 'numbing strategies' so that we can practise super self-care. When we face our fears, we are acting courageously. Courage happens in the mundane. If we observe people in our local community, we can see courage being practised all around us. Just turning up for life every day requires courage, especially when we are prepared to be present.

It takes courage to raise children, to be a loving family member, to be a reliable friend and to go to work. It takes courage to say, 'I want to make a positive difference in this world.' It takes courage to disagree with people, to be willing to take some heat along the way to remain true to our values. It takes courage to admit when we are wrong and it most definitely takes courage to ask for help. The latter two can be the difference between life and death, progress and stagnation. Sometimes it can help to study the biographies of the most extreme cases of those who have demonstrated noteworthy courage (while being mindful not to put people on pedestals). We have enough potential inside of us to demonstrate courage right now. Knowing yourself, and being yourself, is enough.

Grief is a process of emotional healing

Getting in touch with our frozen grief can be a sacred act. Grief work is healing. Grieving allows us to make peace with the past and the present. Grieving helps us to come out of hiding and unravels our masks and false self. We grow stronger and wiser when we get in touch with our original pain. We are no longer chained to our traumatic buried feelings and memories – we are liberated. I learned how to grieve in recovery and with the support of a non-shaming, compassionate, group of fellow travellers. We need to be able to talk about the emotions we are feeling with safe and open-minded people. A good therapist can aid this process. A supportive mindfulness meditation group can be very helpful, too. Ultimately, we can receive support, but no one else can feel our pain and release static, frozen, emotional energy. It is up to us to own our pain and shed our tears.

To feel is to be alive. To be gentle with ourselves and to be vulnerable with others, we have to be willing to fully feel our emotions. I am not referring to self-indulgence. I am stating that, if we are to be fully present in life, to develop emotional maturity and to have a strong sense of self, we cannot afford to numb out. Feeling your feelings may be painful, but you will also experience joyful emotions much more deeply.

Mindfulness

Mindfulness can certainly help to reduce stress, anxiety and depression. Many drug and alcohol rehabilitations use mindfulness to assist in relapse prevention. From my own experience, I know that mindfulness has been incredibly helpful in terms of stress reduction and producing greater clarity. Mindfulness helps us to observe our thoughts without being utterly consumed by them. We can slow down our minds and learn to be at one with our feelings. When we practise mindfulness, we can integrate key areas in our brains and thereby enhance equanimity. We can literally drive connections between the lower regions of our brains (in the brainstem and limbic system) and the prefrontal cortex simply by watching our thoughts without judgement, and feeling our emotions without trying to numb out. We feel liberated when we no longer believe every thought that comes to mind. We feel liberated when we can feel our emotions without panicking. In many cases, we can access a deeper calm in our consciousness and experience what the great sages of the past referred to as *stillness*.

The Vietnamese Buddhist monk and Zen master Thích Nhất Hạnh was exiled from his home country and had to move to France as a result of being a peace activist. During this time Martin Luther King Jr called for Thích Nhất Hạnh to receive a Nobel Peace Prize. I have read and listened to Thích Nhất Hạnh's meditations many times, and he is truly one of the most disciplined meditation teachers in recent times. I feel content with the simplest of things after absorbing his books and guided meditations. His gift has been pointing out the joy in the most everyday things, such as enjoying a glass of cold water when feeling thirsty or enjoying a simple meal. He once said: 'Feelings come and go like clouds in a windy sky, conscious breathing is my anchor.' I have kept this saying in my heart ever since I first read it.

Mindfulness and depression

If a person loses their job, goes through a marriage breakup and becomes physically ill within six months, it would be unnatural for them not to feel angry, sad, low, lonely and frustrated. The problem is that, for many people, low moods can spiral into a full-blown depressive state. Depending on the person's brain chemistry, they may very well be able to recover from the depression by practising mindfulness and other alternative therapeutic methods (grief work, meditation, yoga, etc.). In the last 10 to 15 years mindfulness has been used by medical doctors worldwide to assist in the prevention of relapses into depression. I know of many people diagnosed with both mild and clinical depression who have dedicated themselves to mindfulness practice and cardiovascular exercise and who have shown great improvement in their mental health.

By witnessing our thoughts and being able to identify and label a feeling, we expand our own self-awareness. We can be aware of our awareness and therefore lessen our emotional pain and suffering. When we are prepared to feel our depression, healing takes place. Professor Mark Williams and Dr Jon Kabat Zinn have both done a wonderful job in creating more awareness with respect to mindfulness enhancing mental health. Their book *The Mindful Way through Depression*, written with Zindel Segal and John Teasdale, is well worth reading.

Cultivating a calm mind

Cultivating a calm mind has been possible for me as a result of practising several recovery-based Twelve Step programmes and mindfulness. Although I do not sit down in formal meditation as much as I used to (for over 10 years I sat down to meditate for at least one hour every morning), I now bring mindfulness into my everyday life.

In my early recovery from drug and alcohol addiction, my brain was frazzled. I found it almost impossible to sit still. I realized that if I fidgeted then I could distract myself from feeling my emotions. However, after a year of total abstinence I noticed that quite a few of my fellow travellers in my support group were able to sit still. They had their legs crossed and were relaxed while sharing and listening to others. I realized that I could not do that. I had tremor in my legs, and I needed to continue to move around in my chair. After a while, I became so self-conscious of this that I asked a local member of my support group for help. He suggested mindfulness and gave me a guided meditation to listen to.

This was the beginning of my meditation practice. It took another year or so before I could sit with myself in silence and watch my breath flow in and out of my body. I practised mindful-conscious breathing at home and while travelling to and from my support group. I started to read mindfulness books by the likes of Thích Nhất Hạnh, Eckhart Tolle, Dr Deepak Chopra, Ramana Maharshi, Maharishi Mahesh Yogi and Dr Wayne Dyer. I then explored the Eastern mantra meditations – chanting with beads after reading ancient meditation scriptures from both Buddhist and Hindu texts (the *Dhammapada* and the *Bhagavad Gita*). This particular period in my spiritual practice was very expansive. I dedicated myself to what Twelve Step programmes of recovery suggest: to practise prayer and meditation to improve our conscious contact with a Higher Power of our own understanding. My mind and brain healed tremendously many years later when I did my 'family of origin' frozen grief work. Deep layers of my false self and trance-like states of consciousness dissolved, thereby creating calm in my mind and body. I would highly recommend committing to a meditation group. With the right people, incredible emotional and spiritual healing can take place for both the individual and the group.

If you have read my previous books, you will probably find an Eckhart Tolle quote somewhere in the text. I have resonated with Eckhart Tolle's meditation teachings more than anyone else. His book *The Power of Now* is a classic. I remember reading this in my early twenties, and it helped me a great deal with my spiritual practice. My old friend kindly gave me a copy, which was a wonderful gift. I subsequently bought several copies for my friends. Tolle's gift is that he has been able to use everyday language while teaching how to observe the workings of the human mind. I had heard of stillness prior to studying Tolle's work, but it was not until I read his book that I could identify with what it actually meant. I had had many moments of stillness, but I did not have the vocabulary to explain this to anyone. As I continued to practise conscious breathing, I had deeper encounters of stillness.

Tolle teaches that we can all experience stillness, when we notice the small gaps in between our thoughts. These gaps can last half a second or perhaps a full second. The more we consciously watch our thoughts, the wider the gaps. Stillness feels peaceful and blissful. At times, we may have unexpected moments of stillness. For example, I have had long periods of stillness in my twenties. I did not will this into reality. It just happened. I believe long periods of stillness are an act of grace. Life, even in its most mundane manifestations, looks and feels fresh, vibrant, lush, colourful and beautiful. Eckhart Tolle had a major breakthrough aged 29, after years of severe depression. One day he realized that he was not his thoughts and had a profound spiritual experience. This was the beginning of his spiritual journey, which led him to become one of the world's most authentic meditation teachers. I highly recommend reading his books and watching him talk online.

I always find serenity while spending time by the sea. Recently, my partner and I moved to Brighton and Hove on the south coast of England. It is effortless for me to access inner peace by simply standing on the pebbly beach and watching the waves crash on the sand for 30 minutes or more. I have always been drawn to the sea and the ocean. Standing next to moving water on a gigantic scale lifts my spirits. I recall spending time by the North Pacific Ocean almost every day when I lived in the South Bay, Los Angeles, and on my return promised myself that I would find a way to live by the sea. I spent hours on the Hermosa and Manhattan beaches figuring out what to do with my life (I was two and a half years clean and sober) after my previous career in music had come to an end. My depression and anxiety almost melted away when I walked on the beach.

Learning to relax

It is a myth that relaxation engenders complacency or kills the creative spark. To the contrary, relaxation often creates a better performance at work or even when making love. Rest assured, a sense of urgency can be realized with a relaxed state of consciousness. A sense of urgency is a decision to prioritize something with immediate effect. This can be accomplished while feeling relaxed and calm.

Disproportionate fear and anxiety kill one's potential to live happily, prosperously and peacefully. For example, stage fright does enormous damage to an inspiring actor's career. The number of actors I have met who struggled to perform on stage due to severe anxiety and crippling fear is astonishing. While very mild stress can enhance peak performance, a calm and relaxed state of consciousness produces clarity. Observe the world's finest athletes at the peak of their careers and you will see that they were calm, collected and relaxed while performing.

Public speaking for many people can be a daunting prospect. Although there are many popular courses that claim to teach people how to speak in public without feeling afraid, in my view the best way is to practise public speaking is to utilize meditation. I used to be terribly afraid of speaking to an audience. I got used to speaking to large groups of people as a result of attending support groups. As a writer, I am often asked to lead retreats, workshops and corporate wellbeing events, and, owing to years of practice, I very rarely feel nervous. Whenever I feel a tinge of nervousness, I take several deep breaths and I begin to feel calm. This is due to years of practice and dedication. The athletes and actors I have mentioned who demonstrate a relaxed state of consciousness while performing feel assured in their ability because they have spent thousands of hours practising and dedicating themselves to their craft. This shows how self-discipline and relaxation go hand in hand. No person in her right mind will feel relaxed about talking to a thousand people about a difficult subject if she is not properly prepared. Similarly, no man will feel relaxed walking into a boxing ring if he is not utterly confident in his ability to perform at the highest level. Relaxation, preparation and self-discipline feed off each other.

In the last six years, Rudolph E. Tanzi has become one of my primary meditation teachers. His work on gene expression, the human brain and Alzheimer's has assisted many people worldwide. Dr Tanzi has been able to explain in very simple terms how mindfulness meditation can enhance the human brain. As I became more interested in the science of mindfulness some years ago, I found Tanzi's lectures online and his books (co-authored with Dr Deepak Chora) very helpful. I recommend reading his books *Super Brain*, *Super Genes* and *The Healing Self*.

Your younger self

Symbolically speaking, your younger self (often referred to as your inner child) represents your most vulnerable self. Like many other emotionally wounded people, I find it easier to practise self-compassion when I look at a photo of my younger self. I see an innocent child and feel warmth and compassion for him. By feeling compassion for my younger self, I can practise compassion for my adult self. I have several photos of my younger self. Whenever I am being harsh on myself, I look at these photos and remind myself to relax. Some people can practise self-compassion and reach deep levels of self-acceptance without doing inner child work. We all have different ways to heal. Personally, the inner child work has done for me what 500 self-help and psychology books could not do. The inner child work got me in touch with my frozen grief and started the process of deep emotional healing.

The aforementioned John Bradshaw published a powerful book on inner child work entitled *Home Coming*, which will certainly aid grief work. In fact, all of his books, when studied can bring healing. I regret not meeting Bradshaw in person, although I was honoured when he wrote the foreword to my book *The Kindness Habit* (co-authored with Dr Barbara Mariposa) a year before he died.

For those of us who have reclaimed and reconnected with our younger self, we know all too well how damaging harsh words directed towards ourselves can be. When we realize that we have a duty to re-parent our wounded self, we begin to see the benefit of soothing ourselves through kind words (gentle affirmations) and affirmative action.

Soothing yourself

Self-soothing ourselves can be a part of our super self-care practice. Think of a mother or a grandmother who sings a sweet lullaby to a baby. The melody becomes a sacred transaction between the carer and the baby. In almost all societies worldwide, it is perfectly acceptable for a baby and a young child to be on the receiving end of deep nurturing by a loving maternal figure. The problem occurs when those societies expect the child turned adult to become robotic, unemotional and rigidly self-sufficient. I have witnessed the 'toughest' people soothe themselves by rubbing their chins, necks, the back of their heads or thighs when distressed or irritated. Many people unfortunately attempt to self-soothe by developing damaging addictive behaviours (think of a highly stressed person lighting up a cigarette and inhaling smoke to soothe and temper his nerves). There are healthier ways to self-soothe. We can, for example, practise various deep breathing techniques (mindful breathing, box breathing, etc.), or play music or go for a deep tissue massage or spend an afternoon swimming at a spar club. If we are in a loving relationship, we can ask our spouse or partner to sing to us or we can ask to be held.

Creatures

Between 2010 and 2012 my partner and I lived with and looked after two Labradors (black and gold), three cats, nine puppies, thirty-six kittens and a tortoise. During this time I was going through an emotionally difficult time. I found spending time with our pets a blessing. My stress levels reduced whenever I came into contact with animals. Our pets helped me to slow down my thought-life. They brought a non-human presence into our home, and they were mellow and very sweet. I found that each animal had its own personality and different character traits – I could sense their individual spirits.

While working at a young people's housing association, the company had two therapy dogs visit our residents once a week. We had over 50 residents aged 16 to 26. Conflict among the residents occurred almost every day. However, the therapy dogs always brought a calm presence into the hostel. A raging young woman complaining in the office of a messy roommate would quickly turn her attention to the therapy dog and begin to calm down. Within minutes of stroking the therapy dog, she was much more composed. I always recommend that people, especially children, spend time with animals (unless you have an allergy). There are zoos and farms all over the country which welcome visitors for very little money and sometimes for no fee at all.

Gentleness breaks

Taking gentleness breaks is a good way to practise super self-care. We need to nourish ourselves every day. It is essential to have daily 'me time' where we can enjoy our own company and not feel 'guilty' for doing so. Our 'me time' might be for ten minutes, but for those 600 seconds we can appreciate every moment in time. Some people are on such a tight schedule that the only way they can sit with themselves without inter-ruption is sitting on the loo for five minutes. I recall a British elder statesman saying that sitting on the loo for ten minutes was the only time he had in the day to enjoy his own company, because, as soon as he left the gents' toilets, his PA, office manager, campaign manager and security guard would follow him about until he went to bed at night. The gentleman's toilet seat became a sanctuary for him.

Although I love having a shower, I have started taking more hot baths. This is another way I can rest in hot water with minerals and soaps and let my body loosen up. I can read a paperback, listen to music or just lie in the bath in silence and appreciate the sensations of sitting in a tub of hot, soapy, water. Whenever I have the opportunity, I find it very comforting to light a candle in an old church. Both St Mary's, minutes from Sloane Square, and St James's, minutes away from Hinde Street, are two London churches which have a wonderfully serene atmosphere. Both venues have become my London sanctuaries whenever I am passing by and need a gentleness break.

Gentleness inventory

The following questions may help to bring greater clarity with respect to your own levels of gentleness. If possible, discuss them with a friend or professional.

- How often do you take gentleness breaks?
- What does a gentleness break mean for you?
- Are you hard on yourself for making mistakes?
- Are you too demanding of yourself (a perfectionist) and therefore of others?
- Do you view gentleness and tenderness as being weak?
- How can you demonstrate gentleness in your own life?
- What steps can you take today and this week to be gentle with yourself?
- Are you in recovery from an addiction or a mental illness? If so, are you taking care of yourself? If not, what do you need to do to practise super self-care?

4

Creating authentic relationships

Trust is the most important part of a relationship, closely
followed by communication. I think that if you have those
two things, everything else falls into place – your affection,
your emotional connection.

Vanessa Lachey

A lot of relationships can be saved and rejuvenated with a
willingness to attend couples therapy and/or support groups
and for both parties to be working on their own personal
development. Many unhappy marriages and romantic relationships have come about as a result of two emotionally wounded
people entering a relationship in the hope of being rescued, and
having unrealistic expectations of each other. I have seen this
on dozens of occasions while providing mindfulness training
in residential addiction rehabilitation centres. What chance
do two drug addicts, barely three weeks sober, have in creating
a loving relationship? If an untreated sex and love addict
(someone addicted to falling in love and losing him or herself in
a relationship) and a love avoidant (someone who yearns to love
and to be loved, but constantly pushes his or her lovers away)
have a romantic relationship in the hope of fixing and healing
each other, what is the probability that they will have a healthy,
non-controlling, loving relationship? I know of *one* couple who
met in drug and alcohol rehab, stayed together, got married
and had two beautiful children. They were a rare exception,
however, and they had to work very hard to make it work.

In many cases, the best thing for a long-term miserable
marriage and romantic relationship is to end it. Domestic
violence and sexual and emotional abuse are not acceptable in

any relationship. While I appreciate the institution of marriage, the concept of 'for better or for worse' can keep people trapped in unhealthy relationships. False loyalty, disguised as honouring an oath, is dishonest. A divorce might be painful for a couple, especially if children are involved, but in many cases a stagnant, unhappy marriage can cause greater, ongoing harm. A healthy marriage and long-term relationship can truly be wonderful, but both partners must love each other and work at their relationship every day. All romantic relationships require a lot of work, constant communication and a willingness to listen and to be wrong. Emotional pain is a given in a loving relationship.

Jealousy, possessiveness and power struggles in romantic relationships

Jealousy and possessiveness in romantic relationships often destroy trust and mutual respect. Very often a jealous partner is re-enacting his pain from childhood. If he was emotionally and physically abandoned in childhood, he may be prone to jealousy in a romantic relationship. If a teenage girl was betrayed by her first love, and consequently was emotionally scarred, she may develop jealousy regarding future romantic relationships. Jealousy in a romantic relationship is based on control and possessiveness. A person suffering from jealousy unconsciously believes she is going to lose something or someone she does not own. The partner is afraid of losing her partner. She views him as an object, a possession. No one is a possession of another. The idea that we own or partly own our lovers, even if the sense of 'ownership' is purely emotional, is a delusion which brings suffering in its wake. Jealousy in a romantic relationship is often the body telling us that we need to heal. We have to go deeper in our consciousness and find out what is triggering our suffering. Very likely, an old emotional wound has not been healed.

Some couples will have a problem with power struggles. A power struggle is usually down to competitiveness and old family programming. A couple might try to outdo each other regarding earning capacity, career advancement or social status. Rather than supporting each other and celebrating when their partner has good news, they feel insecure and seek to compete. There can be no real harmony, support or trust in such a romantic relationship. In many ways, the couple are abandoning themselves by staying in such a relationship.

Nasty divorces

Very few people get married hoping to have a vicious divorce. The problem is, when two gravely emotionally wounded people enter a marriage there is a high probability that they will harm each other further. They cannot help themselves. They will constantly trigger each other, play out family of origin scripts and be pulled into age regression. When two people enter a marriage without having addressed some of their past emotional wounds, and are hoping that a marriage is a quick fix to happiness, disappointment and apathy will follow. Bitterness and resentment fuel nasty divorces. It is tragic when children are used as pawns in courtrooms. If financial compensation and revenge become all-consuming, everyone involved will suffer. However, compassion and understanding can turn divorce into a dignified ending. I know of a couple who ended their marriage and gracefully split their assets without lawyers involved. It helped that both parties were in recovery and had to consider their sanity.

A loving relationship begins with you

We have probably heard the saying in lectures, songs, movies, poetry and support groups that *we cannot love another person until we love ourselves*. To love ourselves first must be the basis of all of our relationships if we wish to thrive in this world.

Only you can live in your own body and experience your thoughts and feelings. You can poison yourself with self-neglect and by harbouring ill feeling, or you can nourish yourself with love, a cheerful spirit, eating healthily and living abundantly. You can permit envy and jealousy to spoil your mental and emotional health or you can consciously work on developing emotional intelligence and gratitude. The ancient Buddhist meditation known as *mettā*, loving-kindness, always starts with blessing the individual practising the meditation, before extending love to the world. Loving-kindness meditation is a progressive meditation which begins with you sending warm-heartedness to yourself, then extends to your loved ones, your community, someone you find challenging and then to the world

The difficulty is that it is not possible to be present and to respect our needs if we are still carrying unresolved pain. Many of us are not even aware of our frozen hurt and grief, making self-love even harder to practise. Furthermore, it is impossible to love ourselves if we have not yet accessed our true self. In other words, we cannot love ourselves because we do not know ourselves– our dysfunctional programming, unconscious limiting beliefs and unhealed psychological and emotional pain stifle our efforts.

Practising self-love requires a willingness to be vulnerable with another non-shaming person. An individual's unique experience will determine the actions required to practise self-love. For example, a person severely traumatized in childhood may have to work harder on practising self-love, compared to a person who grew up in a reasonably functional and loving home. The fact is, we all suffer, although some have been more harmed than others. The actions of self-love are often subjective, but a universal approach is to be kind to ourselves. A person may need to be in therapy for two years, whereas the next person may need to be therapy for three months. Another person may join a meditation class and change their eating habits, while another person may need to change their circle of friends.

Creating personal boundaries

Having personal boundaries is an act of love. When we are able to assert a boundary, we are practising super self-care. We are being honest with ourselves about what is both acceptable and unacceptable to us. When we are honest with ourselves about what we wish to discuss with and disclose to others, we are being authentic and honest. This might seem perfectly obvious but a lot of people struggle with asserting personal boundaries due to co-dependency, people-pleasing and low self-worth. Some people may be able to demonstrate their own personal boundaries but they are harsh when asserting them. First, it is essential to know what triggers us and the situations or behaviours that we dislike so that we can begin to develop boundaries. We might, for example, not appreciate someone crowding us, and therefore we might need to move back slightly when that person is talking with us (some people, of course, enjoy the physical proximity of others and so for them this is not an issue). We may not wish to discuss politics or race relations at work, and so it us up to us to have the courage not to engage in such conversations if we know we are triggered by them.

We also need to be mindful of other people's boundaries. We can do this by asking people what is acceptable to them. This is part of building relationships with people. At some point we need to take a risk and *talk* with people. Very often, people who have been severely traumatized will need support regarding developing personal boundaries. For example, I needed a group of men and women to check in with after I asserted a new boundary. I needed honest mirroring and validation from my recovery peer group. I was still emotionally fragile when I started to assert my own personal boundaries. I was afraid of people exploding with rage, which used to be a massive trigger for me. Up until a few years ago angry people frightened me. Today, that has changed as a result of my continuing to take risks by speaking up and knowing that I have a support group behind me.

Overcoming co-dependence

According to Dr Shawn Meghan Burn, a professor of psychology at the California Polytechnic State University, co-dependency is 'a specific type of dysfunctional helping relationship'. In my book *Drug Addiction Recovery*, I have written:

> There are many grey areas when attempting to diagnose co-dependence, because it is very hard to detect unless you are in recovery from co-dependency or are aware of its typical traits. For example, two people can be doing exactly the same thing at the same time, yet one of them is being co-dependent and the other is not. The simplest way to detect co-dependency is by observing the motives behind one's actions. The compulsive need to control people, circumstances and outcomes, in order to avoid feeling one's pain, is what drives co-dependent behaviour.

Typically, a co-dependent relationship is based on a person enabling some sort of dysfunctional behaviour or an addiction. The Karpman Drama Triangle is a simple model that helps us understand one of the classic dynamics in a co-dependent relation. For example, it is extremely likely that a spouse married to an alcoholic will develop co-dependence. His wife's drinking continues to spiral out of control, and so he attempts with every fibre of his being to 'cure her' of alcoholism. He tries to 'manage' her alcohol consumption and thinks of all sorts of ways he can beat alcoholism. He becomes increasingly frustrated and resentful as he realizes that the more he attempts to temper his wife's drinking, the stronger the hold her alcoholism has over her. He burns out and feels at odds with his wife, himself and the world. Having once felt like a 'rescuer' and useful husband, he now blames his wife for his emotional meltdown and becomes somewhat of a victimizer. His wife resents her husband for interfering with her drinking and continues to behave defiantly. The husband who spent years trying to resolve his wife's problems was actually subconsciously trying to avoid having to face his own emotional wounds. This is a clear example of a co-dependent relationship. Another example might be a co-dependent parent compulsively bailing her son or daughter out of financial debt. Essentially, any compulsive enabling behaviour could be a manifestation of co-dependence. I highly recommend reading *Facing Codependence* by Pia Mellody. It is a classic book and will certainly help to provide greater awareness of and insight into this complex behavioural disorder.

Overcoming co-dependence is possible with the help of at least another person who has retired from co-dependent behaviour. There are plenty of strong recovery support groups which address co-dependence, particularly Twelve Step programmes. We need people to mirror back to us our own unconscious behaviours and to observe how people in recovery are facing life's challenges. The key element is to become aware of our own patterns of behaviour and then embark on arresting them, one day at a time. Having arrested co-dependent behaviour, we can then begin to heal our wounds which have been driving us to either play the victim role, the rescuer role or the persecutor role. A good question to remember to ask ourselves before we are about to help someone is: 'Why am I really offering to help this person?'

Overcoming love addiction and love avoidance

Overcoming love addiction is possible, just as it is possible to transcend co-dependence and rebuild a healthy relationship with ourselves and others. Love addiction can manifest in all sorts of different behaviours. For example, some love addicts are addicted to the intensity and infatuation of falling in love. Typically, love addicts will have almost zero boundaries in a romantic relationship and will try to have all of their needs met by their lover. When they realize that they cannot possibly have all of their needs met by their romantic partner (they find this out after the 'falling in love stage' has run its course), they will become disillusioned and resentful and may look for another lover to re-energize them.

Many love addicts fall in love very easily and lose themselves entirely in their relationship. They may neglect their own needs to attempt to satisfy their new romantic partner, hoping that by doing so they will not be abandoned or left for another person. A love addict might very well project fantasies of 'perfection' on to their new lover, only to realize that their 'saviour' cannot live up to such a high ideal. Many love addicts will confuse sex with love and have a deep sense of loneliness and shame. Love addicts are emotionally wounded, shame-based people. The problem is when a love addict realizes by their own admission that they cannot have healthy romantic relationships, they might very well cease relationships altogether, including sex. This is referred to as sex and love anorexia. They starve themselves of sex and hide from engaging in relationships. Therefore, they compound their sense of loneliness and isolation, causing them to retreat from life still further.

Love avoidance is quite the opposite to love addiction. Very often, a love addict will attract a love avoidant and vice versa. Both parties are afraid of being alone and demonstrate self-abandoning behaviour (see Chapter 2). A love avoidant will secretly wish to be in a loving, long-term, erotic relationship but is terrified of commitment. They may very well indeed get involved in a romantic relationship with a love addict, but will find all sorts of ways to suspend the intensity. Vulnerability to a love avoidant is a series threat. They will do everything to avoid revealing their true selves.

When both a love addict and love avoidant feel 'trapped' in their relationship, terrified of being alone but each being triggered by the other, all sorts of dysfunctional behaviour will follow.

When I did a thorough self-appraisal with a recovery mentor at the time, I identified more with being a love avoidant. At the root of my fear of commitment were unaddressed emotional wounds, which thankfully I have been able to resolve. It was by no means easy, and there was a 30-day emotional and physical withdrawal period, which occurred after I decided to stop acting out my patterns. I was attending a Twelve Step programme and fellowship which supported me through this. I could not have done this by myself. I personally know of dozens of love avoidant and love addicts who have completely resolved their issues regarding dysfunctional romantic relationships and have consequently improved their lives. Many people all over the world have healed from love addiction and love avoidance. Here are some helpful tools to address love addiction and love avoidance:

- Be very honest with yourself and examine your patterns in a romantic relationships. Are your patterns of behaviour healthy or dysfunctional?
- Get a recovery mentor or a Twelve Step sponsor who has overcome their love addiction and love avoidance and who is available to assist others.
- Attend at least two support groups a week regarding love addiction and love avoidance. After 90 days you'll start to become much more aware of your addictive patterns of behaviour. Write out your reflections and discuss them with your fellow travellers in recovery.
- Put time aside every morning for meditation, even if it's for just ten minutes. Focus on your breath for a few minutes and ask your brain to make you more aware of

any potential triggers which might otherwise seduce you to act out.

- Be very gentle with yourself. Recovery needs to be a gentle process.
- Saturate your mind with books and talks on love addiction/ love avoidance recovery. Bathe your subconscious mind with new ideas and optimism that you, too, can heal and overcome love addiction and love avoidance.
- Be mindful who you engage with. Make sure the people you are talking to about your recovery demonstrate boundaries and are not going to shame you. A good experienced recovery mentor or Twelve Step sponsor will be able to guide you through this process of attracting non-shaming fellow travellers in recovery.

Relationships inventory

Making an inventory of how our relationships are serving us (or not) can give us greater clarity. See how you get on with this relationship inventory. Create three columns in your notebook and follow the simple guide outlined below with regards to each of your important relationships. After you have made the inventory, discuss your new findings with an emotionally intelligent person. Notice what arises while discussing your inventory.

Person	Feel drained while you are with him/ her or after you have spent time with him/her.	Feel energized, hopeful and optimistic while you are with him/her or after you have spent time with him/her.
Relationship A	X	
Relationship B		X

Creating committed, long-term, erotic relationships

Long-term, loving, erotic relationships take a lot of work, willingness, patience, compromise, deep listening and humility. Many people struggle in long-term erotic relationships, especially after the fleeting 'falling in love' phase has passed. Very often during the first year in a romantic relationship, euphoric and intense emotions, together with high levels of lust, sweep both parties involved off their feet. Excitement, a boost in confidence, and a carefree mood are felt by the couple. This is often described as 'falling in love'. The couple will very often disclose sensitive secrets about themselves, yearning to feel closer to each other. They are high on life and engaged in intense, sexual romance. This can last up to 18 months depending on the couple, but more than likely it will fizzle out after just one year. All too often after 18 months, when hormone levels and feelings of lust having reverted back to normal levels, couples come crashing back down to reality. This can be very disheartening for both parties.

Suddenly, both parties involved begin to character-assassinate each other and find fault at every turn, sex is no longer explosively intense, arguments flare up over trivial things, and buried traumatic emotions are re-enacted and played out in the relationship. In other words, unresolved emotional wounds and trauma contaminate the relationship. A lot of couples break up at this point and then go on to recreate the same pattern with someone new. However, others will recognize their emotional pain and seek couples therapy and/or attend support groups.

The real spark in a committed, erotic, loving relationship, comes when both parties involved have decided to work through their emotional baggage and continue to communicate. This takes a lot of hard work and a willingness to be vulnerable and exposed. If both parties involved are committed, they can develop a deeper and more loving relationship. Their intimacy will grow, and therefore their sex lives will improve, if they continue to work on their relationship *every day*. There will be challenges ahead, but, with respect for each other and a burning desire to stay together, their love will expand and blossom. Even those with the most fractured sense of self, who have been traumatized in childhood, can go on to heal and steadily build a loving long-term romantic relationship with their spouse/partner.

Although I had been working a recovery programme regarding healthy loving relationships (to overcome love addiction and love avoidance), when I met my partner I still had a lot of emotional baggage. I was still prone to mistrust people, especially women, due to past dysfunctional romantic relationships. I was still subject to anger – I would bottle up my feelings for weeks at a time and then randomly explode. I would then have to live with my guilt, as a result of my displays of anger. In hindsight, I was still carrying buried traumatic emotions, which would consequently flare up when I was triggered. It was only when I started to do my deep grief work that I was much less prone to triggers, therefore greatly improving the quality of my relationship with my partner. Until I started to go deep inside my body and access my frozen emotional pain, I was still emotionally living in the past. This was why I was so utterly hopeless in romantic relationships before I got into recovery and started to really check myself.

Being in a long-term, committed, erotic relationship with my partner has helped me develop as a human being more than any therapeutic model, because by being in my relationship I have not been able to hide. My partner has seen many aspects of my human shadow and shortcomings. I have had a constant mirror looking back at me, observing my triggers and generating feedback when appropriate to do so. We cannot hide when we are committed to an honest relationship with our spouse/partner, especially when we have lived with each other for many years. I have had to admit my mistakes promptly in order to sustain trust. Therefore, I have been able to develop emotionally.

In my experience, and having observed many couples over the years, no committed relationship can last without trust. Love depends on trust. Trust is the conduit which love travels through. Without trust, love will remain dormant in human beings. Growing in trust is a gradual process, which occurs one day at a time. Engagement and talking frankly build trust with our partners. We need to be engaged with our partner's needs and wants. We need to feel that our spouse is listening to us. This builds trust.

If you are finding it difficult to stay in a romantic relationship beyond the 'falling in love' stage, it might be worth answering the questions below. Remember to discuss your answers with your spouse/partner if you feel it is appropriate to do so.

- Do you have a problem sustaining a romantic loving relationship?
- Have you ever been in a loving romantic relationship which went further than the 'falling in love' stage?
- Do you still feel good about your romantic relationship after 18 months of being together with your partner?
- What emotions do you feel when your relationship requires great effort on your behalf to move on to mature, deeper love?
- Do you start to feel mistrust, jealousy and rage after 12–18 months in your relationship? If so, where do these emotions come from? Why have they come up now?
- Do you have trust issues?
- Have you previously been betrayed in a romantic relationship?
- Have you betrayed others in your previous romantic relationships?
- Can you discuss your answers to these questions with your partner/spouse in your relationship?
- Are you both willing to work together on creating a deeper love?

If both you and your spouse/partner are serious about evolving together in your relationship, here are some gentle suggestions to consider. First, invest in a fine notepad and a decent pen. This symbolizes that you care about your relationship. Then sit down together and put at least one hour aside to consider the following actions:

- Check in with each other at least every day. Find out how your partner is feeling and what activities they have participated in. Do not do this when one or both of you are distracted. Allocate time specifically to do this. Even if you put just five to ten minutes aside every day, this will be sufficient. Even a text message or an email shows a willingness to engage if, for example, you are on a business trip or a long flight.

- Make a joint inventory together at least every four to six weeks. Discuss different ways to improve your relationship. For example, do you both need to take a break away together? When was the last time you both went on a romantic date together (if money is tight, discuss different ways you can generate more income or creative ways to spend time together). Is your sex life vibrant or does it need a boost? Again, discuss these things with your partner. When making an inventory together, make sure you are both relaxed and can focus on the activity. If you need to put your mobile phone on silent or go for a walk to get some privacy, do so.

- Continue to communicate. I cannot emphasize how important it is to engage and talk with your spouse/partner about any doubts, fears and feelings you have regarding your relationship.

- If you are both in recovery from various addictions or trauma, are you both working diligently on your own individual recovery? It is not a good idea to become completely enmeshed in a romantic relationship. We need to have separate, individual experiences to keep both our lives and our relationship vibrant. Make sure that you both have your own unique support network of trusted, non-shaming people whom you can check in with.

Creating a deeper, mature romantic love

A deeper, mature love with your spouse/partner is much more fulfilling and richer than the act of 'falling in love'. A mature love requires trust, honesty and friendship. This cannot be experienced months into a romantic relationship. Mature love is a process which usually begins to develop after 18 months. It is a practice which can be applied one day at a time. When we are in a deeper, mature love, we can share our joys and sadness with our spouse/partner. We can share our desires and build on those dreams. We can support each other when we are grieving or coming to terms with a loss. We can share intellectual curiosity and laugher and have a strong, healthy attachment figure in our lives. While the beginning of a relationship often produces heightened sexual activity, sex in a mature loving relationship is more intense. People who find that their sex lives are suffering after years of being together will usually find that this has come about as a result of a breakdown in communication (a lack of engagement). Some couples will stay together owing to financial incentives, while others are terrified of being abandoned (both are highly co-dependent relationships). However, when a couple decides to grow together and has put effort into doing so, making love is more natural and has its own rhythm. Here are some questions to ask yourself regarding nurturing a deeper, mature love with your spouse/partner:

- How often do you sit down and talk spontaneously with your spouse/partner?
- Do you have a joint desire/dream you are both working on? Do you have a joint vision? This could be a romantic holiday, planning to buy a home or a new holiday home, or starting up a charity.
- How do you both feel about your home?
- Do you feel that your house/apartment is a home? It is so important to feel good about your home. This is where you and your spouse/partner will have some of the most intimate conversations with each other – where you will make love and disclose your shortcomings.
- Do you feel you both need to sit down and discuss how you can both keep your relationship feeling fresh and vibrant? If so, what actions can you take?

Reconciliation

Reconciliation for many people is very hard to practise. I can understand why. It is hard to think about forgiving people who have harmed us (whether these are real or imagined harms). Some of us were hurt at an age when we could not properly defend ourselves. This makes forgiveness even harder to practise. However, the hardest person to forgive is often ourselves. Self-forgiveness is by no means straightforward; I was able to forgive people who hurt me, especially when I examined my own colourful past, but I was not able to forgive myself for many years. I tried self-empowering affirmations, but to no avail. My own personal reconciliation happened when I started to address my self-loathing. I listened to people in my support group share harrowing stories of self-neglect – I had empathy. Some of my fellow travellers were very hard on themselves for their misdeeds, and I often used to silently criticize them for this. However, I, too, was being hard on myself. My support group mirrored back to me my hypocrisy without telling me I was a hypocrite.

Similarly, I got an awful lot out of listening to my fellow travellers share their experiences regarding reconciliation and self-compassion. They showed me that a new reality was possible. 'If they could forgive themselves, then perhaps I might have a chance,' I used to reflect. Most of the time when I get consumed with resentment, I pray and meditate and talk with a friend about my ill feelings. Sometimes I can address my resentment by writing a self-appraisal, which is often referred to as a personal inventory in the Twelve Step programme of recovery. Additionally, I may need to repeat myself and verbally share my pain until it eventually subsides. Reconciliation is wonderful when it comes from the heart and is sincere. It is, in my view, a spiritual act.

Some people cannot forgive, but even they can find other avenues to bring relief into their everyday life. They can remain active in charitable acts and serve others well, which will bring some comfort and satisfaction in their lives. Ultimately, we are all connected as human beings. We are individuals sharing this planet Earth together at this particular time. We are bound to each other. If I still resent a person, I still resent myself. If resentment towards another person is lifted from me, then I am freed from ill feeling. Whatever I hold on to, compassion or hatred, will affect every part of my being.

Learning to forgive ourselves

It was the carpenter from Nazareth who said: 'Let him who is without sin cast the first stone'. Meditating on this statement has helped me to forgive others and, more importantly, myself. The fact is, we all have our 'stuff' to work through, and I suspect that almost all of us have previously demonstrated regrettable behaviour. Such behaviour is unique to the individual, and so self-forgiveness is a deeply personal experience. While guilt has a role to play in keeping our moral compass in check, excessive guilt and chronic shame do not serve us. Self-forgiveness is one of the hardest things to practise, because we might still be haunted by our regrettable behaviour.

Unless we are sociopaths, we all have a conscience; we can attempt to suppress or manipulate it, but our emotional moral compass operates in the body as well as in the mind. Our bodies will not permit us to take the necessary actions to have loving relationships and prosperous professional and business relationships, if we do not address static emotional energy lingering inside of us. Talking things through with compassionate human beings, and affirming to ourselves that we can learn to forgive ourselves, will gradually heal our emotional wounds. Self-forgiveness is a process and takes time, but the efforts to heal are worth it. If something is disturbing you, write it down in your notebook and discuss it with a trusted friend or a fellow in recovery. This will help to discharge any lingering emotions.

Developing functional professional relationships

It takes time to build some degree of trust with co-workers. To create a decent working environment, we need, at the very least, to understand one another's temperament and respect boundaries. It takes time to figure out what to discuss and what not to discuss with co-workers. It takes patience to understand the style of a new management. The best advice given to me regarding office politics was that 'the walls have ears'. In other words, anything I discuss with a co-worker or manager, no matter how well I get on well with them, will more than likely be leaked to others, accidentally or deliberately.

Common sense certainly helps us to feel comfortable in the workplace. Here are a few tips:

- Try not to character-assassinate your boss to your co-workers, and avoid harsh gossip. Chances are that it will somehow get back to those you have bad-mouthed. If you need to get something off your chest, go outside for a few minutes and call a trusted friend to share your frustrations.
- If your co-workers are turning on a co-worker (most corporate offices *need* to have a scapegoat to keep the patriarchal system operating – all authority-based systems must have an internal and external enemy), avoid getting directly involved.
- Regularly take two to three-minute breaks and remove yourself from the office. Practise mindfulness and deep breathing. Perhaps go for a short walk and distract yourself from your work.
- Remember to keep a balanced, healthy perspective while assessing your co-workers and management.
- If you employ people, remember that, if your employees feel validated and are treated with respect, you will earn their respect and perhaps even their loyalty.

If something is bothering you, you can always ask to talk with a fellow professional when no one else is present and state what is bothering you, but remember that your tone of voice is crucial. By and large, building professional relationships takes willingness, patience and the ability to self-reflect.

All professional relationships are based on a contractual association. Many people often view their office as their surrogate family, and this means that things can often get messy – boundaries are unclear and enmeshment occurs. While it is possible to form friendships from professional relationships, most co-workers will not stay in contact after their contract is terminated. They may add each other to social media accounts, but the effort required to build friendships will not take place. The key thing is to remember to make the best of a temporary professional relationship and to bring humour and amusement to your work life.

Boundary attachment figures versus non-attachment and detachment

The word 'attachment' means different things to me depending on the context. For example, as a result of studying Eastern spirituality, I have learned that it does not serve me well to become attached to an outcome or a result. I need to plan but be open to change or a different trajectory. For instance, we may often get what we want, but our desires manifest in a way we had not dreamed of. In my case, I wanted to have a creative outlet in music, but I ended up writing instead. I still have a creative outlet, but it is not what I previously envisioned. I have written about this kind of non-attachment in my previous books.

In another context, we may need to detach with love from a person or a group of people. We may need to detach with love to protect ourselves – to detach to sustain our personal boundaries. I, too, have had to detach with love; it was painful but necessary. However, in a therapeutic context, we all require human attachment figures. We need to know that we can rely on others to mirror back our thoughts, feelings and actions. We need to have our feelings validated by non-shaming attachment figures who demonstrate healthy boundaries. A loving attachment figure may be a spouse/partner, a close friend, a spiritual teacher, a therapist or a support group. Emotionally wounded people struggle to trust and therefore find it hard to accept when a non-shaming attachment figure offers support. Some people will go through their entire lives rejecting healthy attachment figures and genuine people. This is tragic. While no one can heal another person's emotional pain, we can assist others by listening to them and mirroring their ideas and feelings.

It took me years to attract emotionally available people, and they are my support system. I need this to function, as with them I have the courage to be myself. Similarly, I have become an attachment figure to my partner, family and friends. I can be present, listen and demonstrate healthy boundaries.

The gift of platonic friendship

Almost all successful long-term romantic relationships will be anchored in friendship. However, here we will explore the gift of platonic friendship. The difficulty for many people is that, like all relationships, friendship takes time, energy and effort. When people get married or commit to a long-term, mature, loving relationship and have professional endeavours, it can be easy to convince ourselves that we do not have time for friends. Business and work associates often become many people's way to engage outside of their marriage/romantic relationship. The problem is that business partners and co-workers are a contractual association, based purely on earning money and serving in a company/ charity. As we have covered earlier on in this book, some friendships can bloom as a result of an excellent working relationship, but this is quite rare. Often, when co-workers move on to different companies, their relationships gradually starts to fade.

Another major stumbling block for a lot of people regarding friendship is trust or lack of it. There is always a certain degree of risk when forming friendships, and some people are not willing to be hurt again. They feel safer having professional relationships, because, in some ways, there is less risk of being emotionally hurt, as they are not based on deep, personal intimacy.

For years during teens and early twenties I would find ways to end friendships. I was afraid of intimacy and feeling closely bonded to another person. I thought that my boundaries would be abused, and I would end up being hurt. I much preferred hanging out with different groups of people once in a while. It felt safer. The truth is I was right to be afraid of my boundaries being violated by others, because in my early recovery from drugs and alcohol addiction I did not really have any personal boundaries. I could not hold a sacred space to mirror back my friend's thoughts and feelings, without trying to fix them. However, these experiences were very valuable. They showed me that, although I had got physically sober, I still needed to work on my co-dependency.

Platonic friendship can be truly wonderful if both parties are committed to working on their friendship regularly. Unlike a long-term, committed, romantic relationship, platonic friendships do not need the same intensity and time invested to make them work. We do not have to talk with a friend every day or expect to see them every week.

I have a handful of friends who I mostly met in my early twenties. Like me, they had started to look at their family of origin behavioural traits which they had inherited, and were working on their co-dependency. Some of my friends are not in recovery, but certainly have emotional intelligence and some sort of self-care practice. I cannot have friendships with people who are not practising self-care. It will not work. I need depth, prudence and substance in my friendships. I leave small talk for when I am being introduced to someone for the first time at work or at a social engagement.

I am sure that at times I have irritated my friends or triggered them by something I have said or done. My friends can certainly annoy me at times, but I have tools to deal with my anger and fear. Dealing with envy has been challenging at times, too. I have written in my book *Mindfulness Burnout Prevention* how an old friend of mine and I spent an entire year calling each other to express our good wishes for others, for the express purpose of reducing envy and jealousy in our hearts and minds. It worked, and I am much less envious of others today, if at all. A lot of my friends are intellectually smarter than me, and I feel very grateful to have clever friends. I learn a great deal from them. They help me to sharpen my own intellect and gently prompt me to expand my mind. Some of my friends grew up in very wealthy households (a handful with old famous names), and I have learned to appreciate what their families have contributed to society.

The key is to talk about envy with your friends. A lot of people shy away from this subject in their friendships because it forces people to be vulnerable and honest. If a friend becomes fabulously financially rich, this could cause envy when the other friend is struggling to pay their bills. What happens to the friendship? They will either drift away or talk frankly about envy. They will both need to discuss their fears regarding their friendship. This might feel uncomfortable, but is a necessary part of growing.

There are some things that I will not discuss with my friends and which I keep exclusively for my spouse/partner. This is a healthy boundary. Below I have listed a few things to consider with respect to creating healthy and loving platonic relationships:

- When was the last time you picked up the phone and called your friend? At the very least, sending an email or a text message to check in with a friend is important. Let them know that they are on your mind.
- When was the last time that you and your friend went out together and had fun? When was the last time you belly-laughed together?
- Do you and your friends regularly hang out and talk about your desires and dreams?
- Are you secretly angry, envious or resentful of a friend? If so, is there something you can do about this? Do you have the sufficient emotional and spiritual tools, and a support system to work through your resentment?
- Are you afraid that your friend envies you or is angry with you? Do you have any reason to believe such a thing? Have you discussed this with them?

Who are you?

The more we uncover who we are not and discard our disempowering unconscious behaviours, the more closely we can be in sync with our true, authentic selves. Demonstrating authenticity takes focus and a willingness to be gentle with ourselves. Authenticity is a process. Even those brought up in a very functional and loving home will have to examine their belief system and values at some point in their lives. When we monitor our thoughts and emotions, we can discard what no longer serves us. This takes time and will probably last until we draw our last breath. Authenticity is really a journey of self-discovery. We can make leaps and bounds in short spaces of time, but this is not always the case. Here are some more questions to stimulate your brain:

- Are you really being you or are you playing out family scripts which has been passed down through generations?
- Do you feel you are truly being yourself at any given moment?
- What does it mean to be you?
- What are your values?
- Are your values really yours or are you easily swayed by the opinions of others?

Reflect on these questions and give them some serious thought.

Developing a compassionate heart and mind

There is no fun or joy to be realized if we are holding on to ill feeling towards ourselves and others. When we are consumed with bitterness and resentment, we feel as though life is squeezing us. We end up attracting more people and circumstances which trigger us, and this further aggravates our bitterness and resentment. The cycle continues until we get to a point where we are seriously hurting inside. I have been in this place before, and it is operating in survival mode. Before I created my very first personal inventory, I had resentments galore. I was consumed with envy, jealousy, rage and bitterness. Some of my bitterness was a result of harms done to me, but, as my first recovery mentor explained to me, I was only further injuring myself by holding on to my grievances.

It was a bright and hot sunny day in north-west London, and my mentor and I sat in his back garden while he listened to me share my fears and resentments. I needed to do this to clear my mind, otherwise a risk of a relapse would have been very likely. Additionally, we spent some time in a quiet park in Golders Green, where I disclosed more of my grievances. It was such a relief to air my pain to a compassionate man who did not judge me and who in return shared some of his old wounds with me. I could see that he was serene and was a good person to talk with. As a result of addressing my resentments and fears (there were still hundreds buried in my subconscious which I subsequently addressed years later), I started to feel better about myself and therefore slightly better about the human race. The more I promptly faced my fears and worked hard to eliminate resentment, the more I began to trust myself and therefore others. Gradually, I was able to feel deep compassion for other people because I was no longer distracted by my unresolved pain.

To practise compassion and to have a forgiving streak in one's heart and mind makes life much more pleasant, as we are all social creatures. It is much more likely to create harmony or, at the very least, to reduce fear, if we are prepared to minimize ill feeling towards one another. People will trigger us, and some people can be challenging to be around, but we can draw upon our inner resources and our support network so that we do not have to succumb to resentment and hostility. To have a compassionate mind and heart does not mean that we have to be doormats or lose our integrity. We can be assertive and honour our values, but be mindful not to harbour ill feeling. I have learned to be quite assertive if necessary.

I have written a guided self-love meditation script for you to say out loud, record and play back to yourself. The purpose of this guided meditation is to assist you to direct love inwards. If it helps, you may feel to replay this as and when. If you begin to feel anxious or feel triggered while participating in this exercise, just stop.

Guided self-love meditation

Close your eyes.

Take a deep breath.

Now breathe in for four seconds, hold your breath for four seconds, and breathe out for four seconds.

Be aware that your body is breathing and feel the breath enter and leave your body. Feel your tummy rise, as you breathe deeply in the present moment.

Now be aware of the images on the screen of your mind. Be aware of your thoughts, ideas and concepts. Be the witness of your thought-life. Notice the critical inner voice.

(*Pause for 20 seconds.*)

Now take another deep breath.

Be aware of your thoughts – observe how they come and go – feel your breath sustain you.

Now remember a time when you were hard on yourself. A time when you were cruel to yourself or when you perhaps made a mistake. Feel the feelings of shame or guilt and take a deep breath. Sit with the uncomfortable feelings and continue to breathe deeply.

(*Pause for 20 seconds.*)

Take a deep breath.

Now visualize yourself revisiting your memory. See your wiser self walking towards your wounded self. Sit next to your wounded self and look at him/her in the eyes. Notice how your wounded self feels ashamed and tries to avoid eye contact. Take another deep breath.

(*Pause for 20 seconds.*)

Breathe deeply. See your wounded self looking you in the eyes. Smile at your wounded self and repeat the following words:

I am your future self, and I want you to know that I have forgiven you for your mistakes. I have no ill feeling towards you. I do not hate you, and I have accepted and made peace with your mistakes. I am here to let you know that you are forgiven. You no longer have to hide from life. You no longer have to push good opportunities away which would otherwise expand your life. You no longer need to punish yourself. You have carried enough guilt and shame. It must stop now. I am happy to move on, if you are happy to move. I am happy to clean the slate from now. I am happy for our future to be in sync.

(*Pause for 20 seconds.*)

See your wounded self stand up and embrace you with warm affection. See and hear your wounded self declare, 'I forgive myself – thank you.'

(*Pause for 20 seconds.*)

Now imagine what it would feel like to be free from all of your fears and worries. How would you feel if you could wipe away all of the guilt and shame you have carried for far too long? Imagine yourself feeling comfortable in your own skin, prosperous and serene. Sink into this feeling.

(*Pause for 20 seconds.*)

Hold on to this feeling of directing love inwards.

(*Pause for 20 seconds.*)

Now count from 10 to 0. When you reach 0, take a deep breath and open your eyes.

End recording.

5

Changing the way we look at things

> If you change the way you look at things, the things you look at change.
>
> *Wayne Dyer*

I never had a chance to meet the late Dr Wayne Dyer in person, although his books and audio talks kept me inspired in my early recovery from alcohol, drugs and love addiction. I could relate to Dyer overcoming alcohol addiction and finding solace in spirituality. Let us think about his classic statement given at the top of this chapter, as it can potentially open hearts to a much more fulfilling and happy life.

First, our perception of reality creates our experiences as human beings. If we view the world as a malevolent and hostile place to live in, we will experience such a world. Our brain will home in on all of the darkness in the world. We will therefore attract more of this into our immediate reality. Conversely, if we view the world as a beautiful place to live, albeit with its challenges, our brain will draw upon the amazing love, generosity and kindness taking place around us.

Our perception of reality is primarily based on what we think and feel about the world, regardless of whether our thoughts and emotions are based on a warped ideology. If we do not believe we can build successful professional relationships, or if we view the world as lacking opportunities for us to serve, this will more than likely become what we experience. However, if we challenge our perception regarding opportunity, we will see that, as long as human beings exist, there will always be an opportunity for us to develop professionally and to be of service to others.

Before I worked through a recovery programme, the focus of which was love addiction and love avoidance, I found it very hard to trust women in the context of erotic relationships. I had a handful of female friends from my regular recovery support groups who I bonded with due to our common purpose of recovering from addictive behaviours, but I could not go a step further and allow myself to be vulnerable with a woman if we were sexually acquainted. I had been badly hurt in the past and was left emotionally scarred. In my early twenties, I knew that I needed to get some help regarding romantic relationships. My mentor at the time lived in Santa Monica, California, and guided me through a very emotionally difficult time. I was actually feeling suicidal. He was a cockney Englishman – very to the point, brash and financially wealthy – and had a great understanding of recovery. He suggested that I work through a recovery-based programme around relationships and guided me through the process. Gradually, day by day, week by week, I was starting to heal and my view on taking a risk in a romantic, erotic relationship started to change. I also had to look at my own behaviour and acknowledged that my past behaviour in this area had often been undesirable. Within a year of working relentlessly with my mentor through the recovery programme, I was ready to be in a romantic relationship with a woman. I had gone from a young man who believed it was too risky to get involved with a woman romantically to one who desired such a relationship. Within a year of completing my work around love addiction and sex, I met my partner. *I had changed the way I looked at things, and the things I looked at had changed*. After this spiritual shift, I had the opportunity to guide a dozen men through the programme and assisted them to uncover their unconscious emotional wounds and limiting beliefs regarding romantic relationships. They have all gone on to have healthy, loving and vibrant relationships with their partners, and became more successful in their lives.

It is our unconscious thoughts, emotions, sensations, feelings and beliefs which will paint our reality. The difficulty for many of us is attempting to build a new fulfilling reality if we have experienced something different. When something goes 'wrong' while we are untangling from a co-dependent relationship or creating a new goal, our automatic reaction is to immediately revert back to old thinking and habits. This is where we can take a deep breath, pause and observe our thinking. We can ask the question, 'What am I thinking right now?' From that point, we can dismiss or just let any disempowering thoughts go. Seeing that we have over 50,000 thoughts a day on average, we can chose to hone in our more productive thoughts.

Our best thinking isn't enough to change our lives

My very best thinking led me to a therapist's office weeping and pleading for help regarding my alcoholism at the age of 19. I *thought* I could 'manage' my alcohol addiction, and I failed miserably until I asked for help. My older friends in recovery remind me that I looked like 'death' when I started attending support groups. I was not able to give eye contact, and I covered my eyes with a baseball cap. I had lost significant weight and was frightened to talk to strangers. I was beset with what the programme of Alcoholics Anonymous describes as 'the hideous Four Horseman – terror, bewilderment, frustration and despair'. Similarly, my very best thinking led me to have unhappy, co-dependent relationships. I can go on. The problem was I was dependent on my own counsel. I did not have a support system, let alone a group of sober people to brainstorm with. I just followed my own thinking without getting feedback. The first lesson I learned in recovery was that I needed to check in with sober and wiser people than me regarding my thinking. I still need to do this today. I need feedback from my support system.

The challenge for many people is that they are afraid that they will be shamed if they admit that they do not know all of the answers to their problems. This is usually a result of being brought up in an environment which does not encourage questions and answers, feedback and open non-shaming dialogue. Regardless of how intellectually bright we might believe ourselves to be, we cannot solve our problems without mixing and blending our ideas with others. Most new inventions came as a result of years of feedback from others before the inventor had a breakthrough. For instance, Albert Einstein had mentors, most famously the British ophthalmologist Max Talmey. Tamley encouraged the young Einstein to read books about science and published an account of Einstein's theory of relativity. The most effective people from all walks of life have had a person or group of people they can check in with and exchange ideas. It is important to reflect and receive feedback from wise people, and then meditate on our thoughts. With time we can learn to trust our thinking, after we have changed our subconscious belief system, but we will still require conversations with others to enhance our intellect and stimulate our imagination.

'There is nothing good or bad but thinking makes it so'

It was William Shakespeare who wrote: 'There is nothing good or bad but thinking makes it so.' When I first read this statement in his classic play *Hamlet*, I could not connect with it. However, after a few years of challenging my belief system, and interviewing people regarding personal development, I came to realize that all things are subjective and relative to a different experience. For example, how many times have you changed your perception of a person or an institution or a political party? Perhaps you previously thought you had made a 'definitive' judgement on someone or something, but then your belief system changed. What happened to you? Perhaps an experience caused you to re-examine your thinking. Thinking on a conscious level is relatively straight forward when it comes to challenging behaviour. However, the challenge is being aware of unconscious thought patterns and feelings. We can usually draw something good from something horrible. It may require deep meditation and a desire to challenge our logic and reason, but it is possible to find a different perspective on any circumstance. We are constantly projecting our individual and collective reality with our thoughts, feelings and sensations. We have the power to alter our perception of reality.

Uncovering your unconscious self-image

Our self-image, at a deep unconscious level, is what is driving our behaviour, and therefore our results and outcomes. It is the images we have built over the years about ourselves which manoeuvre us to behave in the way we do. All of the images we hold dearly about ourselves (good or destructive) were planted in our unconscious minds from the day we were born, and by ourselves from the age of three onwards. We were not born with an image of ourselves at birth. We developed such an image by the thoughts and emotions we absorbed from those most closely associated with us. We then compounded the projections of ourselves created by others with the early experiences we had and further crystallized our self-image deep in our conscious mind. As we went along in life, we attracted people, places and things which were in harmony with our self-image. In this context, think of the well-known proverb 'Birds of a feather flock together'. We are attracted to those we resonate with at an unconscious level of awareness. Unless we alter and change our unconscious self-image, we will continue behaving in the same way we have previously. An image of ourselves is really a composite of thoughts, because thoughts are really images. We can alter our self-image by using a faculty in the pre-frontal cortex – the imagination. We will cover imagination and visualization in the next chapter, along with some simple exercises you can use to change your unconscious self-image. If you want to know what your unconscious self-image is, then bravely take stock of your life. Look at where you are regarding all of your personal and professional relationships, your career, where you live and who you spend the most time with. The results in your life are a direct result of your unconscious belief system about who you are. If you desire to alter your results, you must begin to change you, as we will uncover in the next chapter.

How do you view the world?

How we view the world will be our reality, even if our view on life is based on biased and distorted information. It is possible for us to live our entire lives based on poor information and misnomers, thereby stifling our efforts to thrive, and never know any better, unless we make an inventory of our most firmly held views of the world and challenge them. What most of us agree to believe is often based on artificial concepts, which is why the Buddha said: 'In the sky, there is no distinction of east and west; people create distinctions out of their own minds and believe them to be true.'

Answer the following questions and take your time to write your answers in your notebook. Discuss your answers with your recovery or action partner:

- How do you view the world?
- Do you view the world as a dark place with a lack of love and compassion?
- Do you believe it is 'impossible' to have loving and trustworthy relationships?
- Do you believe it is too difficult to attract your ideal romantic life partner?
- Do you believe relationships are too hard to maintain?
- Do you believe you are doomed to live a life without true friends?
- Do you feel there is a lack of opportunity in life for you to express your talents and skills?
- How do you really view yourself?

6

Creating new goals and changing your behaviour

No amount of reading or memorizing will make you successful in life. It is the understanding and application of wise thought that counts.

Bob Proctor

The slightest adjustment in our behaviour can bring a tremendous change in our lives. The difficulty for many of us is that we do not want to feel uncomfortable and at odds with ourselves, which so often happens when we attempt to form a new habit. On average, it takes at least 60 days to form a new habit, both in the mind and body. However, there are times in life when we can make a decision to instantly change our behaviour, but this usually occurs after some sort of tragedy or traumatic experience (for example an alcoholic hitting rock bottom). Sometimes we can decide to change and have all emotional resistance subside, but this is not a usual way to form a new habit.

It is important to understand that it is much wiser to focus on forming a new habit, rather than breaking an old habit. We cannot change the past. The results in our lives today are a reflection of our past thoughts, emotions and deeds. We need to build a new reality (a multitude of new habits) if we are going to change. This is why Buckminster Fuller said: 'You never change things by fighting the existing reality. To change something, build a new model that makes the existing model obsolete.'

For example, it took me almost two years of relentlessly attending support groups before I finally stopped drinking alcohol and taking illegal drugs. The momentum of my alcohol and drug addiction was so powerful that it took a couple of years to have a breakthrough, after a traumatic emotional rock bottom. However, when I got clean and sober in recovery, I stopped smoking cigarettes, but I continued smoking expensive cigars for almost three years thereafter. I was by no means a chain smoker; I smoked a couple of cigars every weekend. Nonetheless, giving up cigars was harder for me to do than giving up smoking cigarettes and cannabis.

We are all unique individuals, and so some of us will be able to form a new habit very quickly while others may need longer. This is especially true when overcoming a destructive addictive behaviour. The good news is that we can form new habits which support a strong recovery from almost any addiction.

Diving deep below the surface of your consciousness

The purpose of this chapter, together with its practical exercises and guided visualizations, is to assist you transcend and change your unconscious and subconscious beliefs, feelings and behaviours, so that you can begin working on your healing emotional blockages. As we have uncovered throughout this book, most of our problems are a result of old family of origin and societal mental and emotional programming, at a very deep subconscious level. In order to make a big change in our lives, we will have to dive deep below the surface of our awareness and begin to alter our programming. This takes commitment on our behalf. Changing years of unconscious habits and warped perceptions of reality will not happen immediately, but we can begin the process immediately.

It was Carl Jung who said: 'Until you make the unconscious conscious, it will direct your life and you will call it fate.' The unconscious emotional wounds and fears we hold on to are preventing so many of us from thriving and enjoying our lives.

Think of the subconscious mind as a giant iceberg. The tip of the iceberg might be large, but it is tiny in comparison to what lies below. The tip of the iceberg in this metaphor represents your conscious mind, and below the iceberg represents your subconscious mind. The more you continue to challenge your everyday thinking and perceptions of life, discuss your reflections with others, and listen to how others are living their lives in comparison to yours (listening to people who, unlike you, have already had breakthroughs in their lives), the more you can consciously challenge your subconscious ideas. The more you practise asking questions, the easier it will be to 'make the unconscious conscious'.

A spiritual practice

Almost all of the world's great sages throughout human history have suggested that we are spiritual beings having a human experience. In my own view, I too, believe that there is so much more to us than our bodies. I believe we are each a spiritual being living in a human body, equipped with a powerful mind. The very essence of our being is non-physical. Spirituality is really profound self-awareness. We have the ability to be aware of our thought-life and our emotions, and we can direct our bodies to create and build our dreams.

In recovery, it is essential to have a spiritual practice. For some people, this means chanting and praying daily. Others may meditate daily. Some people will find peace and tranquillity in a church or temple. Being outside and at one with nature enhances many people's spiritual lives. The amazingly wonderful realization of having a spiritual practice is that it is not rigid. There is no dogma or theories set in stone. A spiritual practice leaves room for us to reflect, challenge and evolve. Having a spiritual solution for an addictive behaviour has proven to be highly effective, as demonstrated in the Twelve Step movements.

If I draw upon my personal experience both pre-recovery and in recovery, I cannot be effective in this world without a spiritual practice and a strong connection with a higher consciousness. Tools such as visualization and affirmations have only really produced desirable results after I addressed my fears, resentments and trauma; I needed to release unconscious toxic energy so that new ideas charged with a higher consciousness could flow through me. In other words, altering my consciousness comes before utilizing mindset methods. I cannot change my vibrational frequency alone by using mindset tools. It is my spiritual practice which will produce the power I need to thrive.

Expectations

There is a saying that 'expectations are premeditated resentments'. However, expectations can be both empowering and destructive. For example, I used to have incredibly high expectations regarding my professional goals which were simply not plausible at the time. I did not have sufficient systems in place or a reliable support system. I made demands on myself to be incredibly productive, while battling with alcohol and drug addiction, depression and frozen grief. Even though I had moderate success in my DJ career, I fell into a deep depression which made it very hard to get motivated. It was very hard for me to sustain positive visibility (see Chapter 3).

When I got sober, I wanted to instantly have as much clarity and serenity as my fellow travellers in my support group, who had been clean and regularly meditating for over a decade. My expectations were not properly thought through and came from an arrested emotional development and mystification. I eventually reached ten years in recovery and realized a deep serenity and inner peace. However, it took years of willingness and painstaking effort to do so. Fifteen years later, I have learned to get some perspective on my expectations.

If a person decides that she wants to learn how to master playing the piano, then this is certainly possible. This intention is based on a plausible high expectation. The time she can commit to practising and listening to great pianists, and other factors such as heath, will have an impact on how quickly she can play like Frédéric Chopin. However, if the person wanting to master her craft is unwilling to put in the effort and hopes to cut corners, then her expectation is unrealistic and destructive. She will become resentful because she has put herself in an unrealistic situation.

If we study all the ground-breaking achievements which were formed with high expectations, we see that the tide was on their side and plenty of thought and consideration was applied to the task at hand. When Bill Wilson met Dr Bob and therefore co-founded Alcoholics Anonymous (and the recovery movement as we know it), the groundwork had been done years beforehand by the Oxford Group, the likes of Carl Jung and recovering alcoholics in the USA. Humanity was finally ready for a worldwide, proven solution to alcoholism and addictive behaviours. It was mighty bold of Bill Wilson and Dr Bob to dream of arresting alcoholism worldwide, but their dream has had a deep impact on the lives of tens of millions of people ever since.

Maria Montessori became the first female medical doctor in Italy. She had such an impact assisting disempowered children that she had to leave Italy, because Mussolini viewed her liberal ideas as a threat to fascism. The Montessori movement which helps to nurture small children in a non-shaming and effective way was only possible because Dr Montessori had a bold plan in her mind. She had many detours but, with a team effort, managed to change the world.

Your human needs and wants

Our human needs, when examined carefully, build a psychological, emotional, spiritual and physical infrastructure that enable us to live a wholesome human life. When our human needs are met, we feel confident that we can meet life's challenges. Conversely, when our human needs are not met, we feel disempowered. If we are people-pleasing and not prioritizing our needs, we will resent ourselves and others. The problem for many emotionally wounded people is that they do not know how to have their needs met, and so they turn their attention to their wants, which are often a way to temporarily numb out. Marketing forces bank on selling many of their products to extremely needy people. They know that they can target a specific demographic, on the basis of the 'Buy this product and you'll be OK'. The good news is that emotionally wounded people can learn to get their human needs met in adulthood.

We all need to be loved and to love. We all need to realize our developmental human stages. We all need to grieve and process our losses. We need some sort of spiritual (though not necessarily religious) practice. We all need to engage in fulfilling work – to be of service to others in our own unique way. We require friendship and fellowship, and we need to be validated. Some people need to be employees, and some people need to be employers, depending on their temperament and inclination. Personally, I require a nourishing and healthy diet (I eat an entirely plant-based diet), daily prayer and meditation, rest, exercise, intellectual stimulation, fellowship, good music, challenging books to study (on recovery, history, politics, science), and time with my partner, family and friends. I need sufficient sources of income so that I can be fully self-supporting and enjoy my life. I need to travel and invest in new creative projects. Because I am human, I sometimes miss the mark and neglect some of my human needs, but there are plenty of days when I feel whole.

Below are some questions to help you access where you are with respect to your human needs and wants. It might be worth discussing your answers with your spouse/partner or a group of friends.

- What are your needs?
- Are you getting your needs met?
- Do you feel uncomfortable getting your needs met (for example asking for what you need from your spouse/partner, employer or a friend)?
- What do you need to do to get your needs met?
- What are your wants?
- Do you feel guilty for your desires and wants? If so, why is this?
- Do you feel uncomfortable when discussing your wants and desires with people? Is there a sense of shame or an emotional blockage in this area?

Hamartia

Emotionally wounded people have a much harder time understanding the necessity of failure, compared to those who have a healthy sense of self. An emotionally wounded person will feel as though *they* are a failure after experiencing a defeat. Unresolved emotional pain flairs up whenever there is a failure to achieve a goal. Failure can be so triggering that an emotionally wounded person might immediately numb out, isolate or have a complete meltdown.

The verb 'to fail' is related to the concept of sin. The Greek word for 'acts of sin' used in the New Testament is *hamartia*, which is derived from the verb *hamartánein*, meaning to 'miss the mark'. *Hamartia* (failure) thus describes an action, not a person. Just because we fail, it does not mean that we are failures. Without missing the mark, we cannot learn and grow. Therefore, failure is just as important as success. Neuroscientists have proven that when we learn from our defeats, as a result of our mistakes, we develop new neural pathways in the brain, and become smarter and stronger. We all experience failure; it is just that we live in a world which demands rigorous perfectionism and flawless achievement. Tragically, the world shames people for failing. The illusion of perfectionism dominates most commercial marketing. The good news is that I have noticed that people are becoming less embarrassed to talk about their defeats, especially on social media (this is one of the positive aspect of social media).

To dream a dream

As human beings, we need to dream of new realities. To dream and to bathe in your heart's desire unleashes enthusiasm and a new lease of life. The problem many people have is that they find it hard to manifest their dream. They fear taking a risk and being visible, just in case 'things go wrong'. Many people may be able to muster some physical energy to begin working on their dream, but within months their enthusiasm fizzles out. They part with their dream and settle for what they *think* they can achieve. A lot of people become despondent and live with apathy after meeting with seemingly unsurmountable obstacles. They become rigid, cynical and resentful. I understand this personally. I have been through very rough patches in my life, which stifled my will to dream and live. When we are in such a low emotional state, we need human aid. We cannot pull ourselves out of grave emotional pain without warm-hearted human relationships. It is our connections with people which will inspire us again.

Paintings, films and songs, which are often credited with reviving people's inspirational thoughts, are by-products of human relationships. When we dream of a vibrant and fulfilling reality, we re-energize ourselves. To dream is to uncover the un-manifested – a reality which lies dormant and is beyond this world, but which can be experienced in this world. By this I mean we have to hear a song in our minds, and dream of recording a song, before we can actually hear it on a sound system. We need to dream and visualize a picture before we can paint it and therefore bring it into the physical world. This is why Vincent van Gogh said, 'I dream of painting and I paint my dream.' Similarly, Martin Luther King, Jr stated that he *had a dream*, during his iconic speech on the Lincoln Memorial in 1963. He inspired people to use their imagination, knowing that inspiration flows through people who dream of creating a better world. To dream connects us with a higher level of awareness, beyond the five senses.

An excellent exercise is to draw or paint a picture of your dream. This helps to expand your imagination and rewire your brain. This exercise is more effective when done with two people. When you have a physical image of your dream, spend a few minutes every day looking at this picture, and sink into the feeling of already attaining it. Naturally, no dream will manifest without effort on our behalf, but putting time aside every morning and evening to feel in possession of your dream will begin to rewire your brain and alter your unconscious mind. Within a relatively short period of time your body will respond and act accordingly. I will expand on this shortly. In the meantime, do you have someone who can join you in this exercise? Answer the following questions to activate your dreams:

- What is your dream?
- What do you wish to create?
- What does this desire look like?
- What colours do you see in your dream?
- Who is in your dream?
- How does this dream make you feel?

Use your imagination

As human beings we have been blessed with the gift of imagination. We can use our imagination to create a new environment and change our lives. Our imagination can help us to visualize our future selves living more abundantly, and serving others more effectively. We can actually create images in our minds and manifest them in this world. We are the most successful creatures on earth and much of this is to do with our imagination – the ability to change our environment whenever we choose.

When I got sober my friend showed me a quote on his laptop by Albert Einstein. It read: 'Imagination is more important than knowledge.' It sounded good at the time, and I could intellectually grasp his statement, but it did not emotionally connect with me until many years later.

Let's consider Einstein's statement for a moment. It is our imagination which helps us to access the *unknown* – realities we can access from the mystery of thought and desire. This is what Maria Montessori did when she had a vision to create a global movement to aid and support children to find their true selves, and to guide them to develop emotional health. Today we know that the first three years of life program me a child, and this more often than not dictates the direction of the child's life (although as adults we can rewire our brain by using our imagination and creative thought). Dr Montessori intuitively understood the importance of nurturing children from a very young age so that they can thrive. She was a genius in her own right – a true visionary. Many great scientific and philosophical minds, from Aristotle to Newton and Darwin to Einstein, all used their imagination.

The problem is, many people are using their imagination in a destructive way. Rather than imagining themselves living successfully, they allow their unconscious programming to dictate their future. They are stuck in the past, imagining themselves living a hard life. If they have untreated mental and emotional illness and addictions, this makes it even harder for them to change their lives. Those suffering from mental illness and addictive behaviours must do some emotional recovery work if they are going to be in sync with the higher levels of their imagination. I needed to apply several Twelve Step programmes and deep-feeling grief work before I could command my imagination to serve me. Prior to emotional grief recovery, I was still stifled in my efforts to get in harmony with my imagination. A person with complex PTSD, or PTSD, or frozen grief will need to take this into consideration when they begin to consciously harness their imagination. When we begin to consciously change our lives, we will have to face our fears and feel our emotional pain, before we can effortlessly use our imagination. There is no other way round this. In many respects, I was powerless over my unconscious and subconscious limiting beliefs and frozen grief for many years, despite the fact that I was sober and making some progress in life.

Our imagination can help us to transcend our everyday habits and create a new world for us. Most of us are repeating the same everyday habits and thoughts. The more we repeat the same thoughts and behaviours, the more they become wired in our brains and bodies. The past repeats itself. This is why it can be incredibly difficult to change our ways in adulthood. However, our imagination gives us an opportunity to see ourselves living differently. We can dream a desire, see it, feel it, and begin to take action. It is our imagination which can help us to change course in our lives. We do not have to succumb to the past – we have a choice to change if we are willing to take action, and get some help. Answer the following questions to activate your imagination:

- How often do you deliberately use your imagination?
- Do you find it hard to hold on to an image in your mind?
- Do you find it difficult to use your imagination?
- What do you desire? Can you use your imagination to dream your dreams?
- How do you see yourself?
- Can you dream a more wholesome version of your future self? If so, what do you look like? How do you walk? How do you behave? What clothes do you wear? Where do you live?

Use your brain to thrive

Think of how hard it was to learn how to tie your shoelaces when you were a child. This was a big deal at the time. However, after plenty of practice you finally managed to tie your own shoelaces. Similarly, think about how hard it was to learn to ride a bike or drive a car. This might have been a daunting prospect at first. However, as a result of your persistence, within a reasonably short period of time you succeeded. If you have been driving a car for a while, you will notice that you automatically drive without much conscious thought. Your body just takes over when you close your door and start up the engine. Your unconscious mind takes full control, but it was *you* who programmed your unconscious mind to do so. You must have imagined yourself driving unconsciously before you drove a car for the first time. Similarly, you did the same when learning to speak or understand a language. People readily accept we can change our behaviour and therefore change our lives when it comes to everyday tasks such as learning to read and write, having a bath or a shower, walking and talking. However, when it is suggested that they use their brain to create a more fulfilling life, doubt creeps in for a lot of people. Their unconscious programming has convinced them that, by the time they have got to a certain age, they should accept their lot and hope for the best. They have lost the confidence they once possessed in early childhood to explore the world and take new risks.

The fact is we can use our brain to change the way we live, from moment to moment, one day at a time. Such a practice is referred to as 'neuroplasticity'. We can deliberately rewire our neural pathways, as a result of thinking and imagining new ways to live, followed up by immediate action. According to Dr Brooklyn Storme:

> The function of a belief is in part to help us make sense of the world around us. It creates a filter for our brain to receive, store, interpret and recall information picked up from the world around us by our senses and it automates the way our brain processes information. In order for a thought (which occurs in the conscious mind) to become a belief, it must be repeated. It's this repetition that allows a neural pathway to be created.

In my *HuffPost UK* blog I interviewed one of my mentors, the aforementioned Rudolph E. Tanzi, regarding rewiring the brain to create a better life. (Dr Tanzi wrote the foreword to my book *Drug Addiction Recovery*, which I recommend to those recovering from drug addiction or those closely associated with drug addicts.) According to Dr Tanzi:

> Your brain brings you your world. Your entire world is brought to you by your brain, so how your brain is wired really defines the world you are living in. If you take time to observe what your brain is bringing you, driving connections between these regions, that brings integration – integration of mind and brain is what will then optimise the wiring of your brain to bring you the world that you will most enjoy and give you a good life.

Similarly, Dr Dan Siegel has written on the website psychalive.org:

> Contrary to what we used to believe we now know that the brain is open to change throughout the lifespan. And what some people don't realize is that not only can the brain

change, but we can learn to use the focus of the mind to actually change the connections in the brain itself.

Here we have two towering giants (Dr Tanzi and Dr Siegel) in the neuroscience field clearly stating that we can change our lives by rewiring the brain. How wonderful!

In the programme of Alcoholics Anonymous it is written:

> On awakening let us think about the next twenty-four hours ahead. We consider our plans for the day. Before we begin, we ask God to direct our thinking, especially asking that it be divorced from self-pity, dishonest or self-seeking motives. Under these conditions we can employ our mental faculties with assurance, for after all God gave us brains to use.

The AA programme, first published in 1939, is clearly suggesting that with spiritual practice we can work with our brains and use our mental faculties to create new plans and approach the day with a sound moral compass.

Going beyond your five senses

The difficulty many people have when trying to form a new habit and to visualize their future self is that they have been conditioned to operate from their five senses: hearing, sight, smell, taste and touch. Very often, they will look at their immediate reality and become frustrated with how things currently are. They decide that things are not improving fast enough and give up on forming new behaviour and habits. It is essential to understand that imagination is a higher mental faculty and does not operate within the five senses.

When you imagine yourself having great friendships, an amazing relationship with your spouse/partner or a future spouse/partner, or excelling in your line of work, your five senses will suggest that this cannot be. Your five senses cannot fathom the wonders of your imagination, let alone intuitive thoughts and hunches. This is where discipline comes in. When we doubt ourselves, it is up to us to temper our five senses, remember our intention to change, and call upon our imagination to raise our energy and vibrational frequency. If we are members of support groups, we can call upon our fellow travellers to remind us to persist as we strive to change our behaviour. While is important to appreciate our five senses, we also need to understand that there are higher elements we must use if we are to make a conscious breakthrough in our lives.

Anchor the present with a newfound belief in yourself and your dream

For years I had flashbacks of traumatic memories and emotions going back decades. As a result, it was very hard for me to emotionally connect with my affirmations and visualization practice. I could intellectually state what I wanted to do to improve my life, and I could build a vision in my imagination, but I was not able to emotionally connect; I was still numbing out. I was in the midst of untreated process addictions and unresolved trauma and grief. Thus, flashbacks continued.

A year after I had addressed my emotional wounds from the past, I had a new enthusiasm to thrive. I could emotionally connect with my visualization practice. Then I noticed that images from my morning and evening visualization practice appeared in my mind randomly throughout the day. The images were flashes of my desires. Just as I had had traumatic flash-backs from the past, I started to have emotional flashes from the un-manifested. I was anchoring the present moment with a newfound belief in myself and my dreams. The more I practised emotionally based visualization, the more I had thoughts which reflected the desires that consumed my mind throughout the day. My everyday emotional state soon matched my dream of my future self. I spend two hours a day on average visualizing and, more importantly, to emotionally connect with my goals.

I know that, by doing so, I am compelling my mind and brain to deliberately attract people, places and things into my reality to assist me in turning my dream into a physical fact.

Right now in this very moment you can decide to create a more fulfilling life and begin to imagine how this would feel. By doing so, your behaviour will be much more in tune with your dream. You will be creating a belief within yourself that you can achieve your goal.

Change you

Most people are trying to change the outcomes in their lives, rather than changing themselves as a person. They want to have meaningful, loving and trustworthy relationships, generate more capital, get physically fit or set up a business, without truly putting in the effort to rewire their brains and change their subconscious programming. This is putting the cart before the horse.

Consider the following. A woman looks in the mirror and realizes she desperately needs new clothes. She looks at her reflection and tries to change it without actually changing her clothes. You would have to agree that this is an impossibility, but this is what most people are doing in their lives. Rather than examining their behaviour and belief system, they are trying to change their outcomes and results. Therefore, nothing really changes. They are repeating the same behaviour and expecting to get different results, only to end up with the same disappointing outcomes.

I, too, struggled in this area for many years. I *thought* I had to change my results for my results to change. I was brought up to believe this by my family of origin, teachers at school, friends and society. It was in my early twenties that I had heard of the concept of focusing on changing behaviour rather than wasting time trying to control results. Even after hearing this at hundreds of Twelve Step meetings over several years, I could only understand this concept intellectually – I could not apply it. I was lacking praxis. According to the *Oxford English Dictionary* praxis means 'A way of doing something; the use of a theory or a belief in a practical way.' After years of listening to this concept of *changing behaviour to change results*, as I continued to deliberately rewire my brain, it started to make sense at a deep emotional level. When we emotionally connect with a statement, a concept or belief, we have actually connected a statement, concept or a belief deep within the body. Therefore, a 'shift' has taken place. Our behaviour will change, and therefore our results and outcomes *must* change.

We can only change our thoughts, beliefs and behaviour – the results and outcomes in our lives are not our business. If you were spiritual or religious, you might word it like this: 'We take care of the actions and God takes care of the results.' From a scientific point of view, we might say: 'Our thoughts, feelings, beliefs and actions are the *cause*. The results are the *effect*.'

How often do you question and evaluate your belief system with respect to what you believe you can achieve?

Your outcomes and results are a reflection of your deep entrenched belief system. An important exercise to do is to honestly examine the results in your life regarding your personal and professional relationships, your career (or lack of one), your income and lifestyle. Make a personal inventory of your 'stock' and be honest. This might cause discomfort and emotional pain, but it is absolutely necessary if you wish to change your behaviour and therefore change your life.

Do this exercise with your recovery partner, or an excellent therapist or your spouse/partner – someone who understands why you are taking a self-appraisal (they must be non-shaming and encouraging). An experienced, non-shaming, friend, mentor or support group can be invaluable while working towards self-love and self-acceptance.

The emotional discomfort or unease which is stirred up as a result of a fact-finding inventory needs to be felt, validated and processed with a person who wants us to succeed. When we *feel* the extreme discomfort generated by a 'shame grenade' fully, we heal a wounded part of ourselves which otherwise would have remained dormant in the body. We need to feel our shame and embarrassment which we have been in denial of before we can move on and establish new behaviour.

By feeling our shame-based emotions, we are driving connections in the brain – the prefrontal cortex, limbic system and the brainstem. The prefrontal cortex is a channel for imagination, higher thought, reason, complex planning, empathy and compassion. The limbic system is responsible for our emotions and short-term memory (both the hippocampus and amygdala, which acts as a 'warning bell for danger' and stores traumatic memories and feelings, reside in the limbic system) as well as many other important tasks. The brainstem is responsible for your breathing, heartbeat, sex drive and the infamous 'fight, flight, freeze and faint'. When you begin to change your thoughts and beliefs and begin to attempt to change your behaviour, your brainstem and limbic system will produce chemicals in the body, which will act as a fire alarm in the body. Feelings of fear, shame and even terror will be felt throughout the body. This is perfectly natural. When we fully understand that this is a natural part of the process of rewiring our brains, we can continue to persist, knowing that within a reasonably short period of time, new behaviour will be established.

We need to come out of hiding so that we can thrive. If we wish to symbolically flush out frozen shameful feelings about ourselves and our lives, we need to be at one with our emotions until they pass. In 2012 my book *The Mystery of Belief* was published, which was written to help readers to develop self-belief from scratch. Although it is a quick read, the ideas in the book will certainly assist you to stay on track while changing your subconscious beliefs.

Answer the following questions with your collaborator. The key thing is to be honest with yourself and another person, and steadily make improvements, one at a time. We are never going to be 'perfect', and so progress is the watchword.

Romantic relationship

- Do you trust your spouse/partner?
- Do you still love your spouse/partner?
- What is your sex life like?
- Does your sex life need to improve?
- When was the last time you both went on holiday together?
- How often do you do things together?
- Do you fight or argue more often than enjoying each other's company?
- Do you resent your spouse/partner?
- When was the last time you both made an inventory of your life and created new goals and plans together?
- What needs to improve in your relationship with your spouse/ partner?

Personal relationships

- Describe what your personal relationships are like.
- Do you trust your friends?
- Can you have honest, non-shaming, deep conversations with your friends?
- Do your friends encourage and support you?
- Do you regularly feel drained after spending time with your friend(s) or do you often feel more yourself after leaving their company?
- Are you afraid of your friends turning on you if you make the changes you need to make in your life in order for you to live happily and abundantly?

Your career

- Do you have a career or are you just working in a job for the sake of having a job?

- Are you stuck in your career? If so, why do you *think* you are stuck?
- Do you love your career?
- What can you do to improve your prospects to advance (if you wish to advance) in your career?
- What bothers you regarding your career?
- Are you prepared to ask for help and support to change your approach so that you can enjoy your career?
- Are you satisfied with your salary?
- If you own your own company, are you happy with your employees? Do you trust them?
- How can you move your business forward?
- What needs to change for your business to succeed in the next three to five years?

Your health (mental, emotional and physical)

- Are you honestly looking after your body?
- Are you getting the recommended seven to eight hours sleep most nights?
- What are your eating habits? Do you consume junk food more than healthy meals?
- How often do you exercise?
- What do you consider sufficient exercise?
- Do you like yourself?
- Do you feel angry and afraid most of the time?
- What emotions are you feeling most of the time?
- Do you suspect you have a mental illness? If so, have you sought professional help? What steps have you taken to receive help?

A super self-care inventory

The following questions have been taken from my 'Super Self-Care' seminar. I ask my clients to answer the following questions and to share their answers in a group. I ask clients not to directly comment on people's answers but to keep the focus on their own answers. They gain value from listening to themselves share their answers out loud. Similarly, they gain value by listening to other people without commenting or interrupting. The workshop therefore becomes a safe place with boundaries. It is well worth discussing these questions with another person, as previously recommended. (If some of the questions are similar to previous questions asked in this book, please keep in mind this is to assist you in thoroughly access your subconscious beliefs.)

- What does self-care mean to you?
- What practical steps can you take to enhance super self-care in your personal, professional and social life?
- What do you feel is stopping you from taking practical steps to enhance your personal, professional and social life? For example, a person might shy away from social gatherings as a result of the fear of being judged (the fear of visibility).
- How can you enhance your mental, emotional, physical and spiritual wellbeing?
- What does fun mean to you, and how can you bring more fun and joy into your life?
- How often do you put time aside to rest your body and therefore practise quality downtime?
- If you find it hard to put some time aside to rest properly, what steps can you take to improve downtime?
- Can you think of at least one person (ideally two people) who can support, encourage and hold you accountable with respect to enhancing self-care?
- What is self-compassion?
- How can you demonstrate self-compassion in your everyday life?
- Which areas in your life are you finding stressful?
- What practical steps can you take to reduce stress?
- What is your vision for your life?
- What steps can you take to move forward?
- What thoughts and beliefs about yourself might be blocking you from realizing your vision?
- What steps can you take to transcend your limiting beliefs about yourself and what is possible to achieve?

- Do you feel stuck in your life? If so, in what areas do you feel stuck?
- Are you feeling depressed?
- Are you stuck in your career? If yes, why do you feel stuck? What are your options going forward?
- Are you working in a toxic working environment? What steps can you take to attract a more rewarding job or generate another source of income?
- Do you need to make improvements regarding your financial affairs? If so, what practical steps can you take today to make a positive change?
- Do you have regular suicidal thoughts? *If the answer is yes, please visit a medical professional as soon as possible.*
- Do you feel stuck in your recovery?
- What can you do to keep your recovery vibrant? For example, a person may attend a retreat or a recovery convention to give them a mental uplift.
- Do you have a fun, creative outlet?

If you have not answered the previous questions and discussed them with a friend or in a non-shaming support group, go back and answer the questions. If you felt a strong resistance to *answer* the questions above or decided that you did not have the time to do so, this could be your subconscious programming stopping you from changing your behaviour. Think about this for a moment.

Decide what your primary goal is

If you have answered all of the questions in this chapter and book and discussed them with another person, now is the time to decide to focus on a particular dream or desire you would like to turn into a goal. A goal is really a dream with a deadline. When we decide to put a time frame on our dream, we are much less likely to procrastinate. We feel a sense of urgency and therefore move into action.

Write down your goal in your notebook, using the present perfect tense ('I have done so and so') as though it is already accomplished. By doing so, you are in the process of creating a deep belief that you are in harmony with your dream. Once your body believes this to be true, your behaviour must change. In psychology, this is called self-suggestion or autosuggestion.

New ideas to create your dream will appear in your conscious, mind and your prefrontal cortex will lead the way. If you are spiritually nourished and operating from your true self, you will find it much easier to manifest all sorts of wonderful things in this world, rather than purely relying on your own will power. Here is an example of how to write out your goal in the perfect tense:

> I am grateful now that I have attracted my dream spouse/
> partner. I have dedicated time and effort every day to grow
> as a human being, so that I could match and resonate with
> my dream spouse/partner.

Read your goal out loud at dozen times a day and put time aside first thing in the morning, afternoon and evening to read out your goal and imagine you have already accomplished your goal. Sink into the feeling of what it would feel like to accomplish your goal. Put at least five minutes aside in the morning and again in the afternoon, and again in the evening to get emotionally and physically in sync with your imagination. I often put 20 to 30 minutes aside to do this every morning and evening. The idea here is to emotionally and physically convince yourself (your mind, brain and body) that you are in harmony with your vision. Remember that your brain creates your reality. Utilize neuroplasticity and your imagination to manifest your goal.

Way back in 1937 the US self-help author Napoleon Hill stated:

> If you repeat a million times the famous Emil Coué formula,
> Day by day, in every way, I am getting better and better,

without mixing emotion and FAITH with your words, you will experience no desirable results. Your subconscious mind recognizes and acts ONLY upon thoughts which have been well-mixed with emotion or feeling.

A gestation period

While working towards your primary goal, it is important to understand that there is a gestation period. In other words, there is a time for sowing and a time for reaping. When you decide to make a positive change in your life, perhaps to improve your relationship with your spouse, or to attract a spouse/lover, or to thrive in your career, you have planted an idea (the equivalent of a seed) in your mind. You will need to feed your idea with the feeling of already manifesting your goal to penetrate your subconscious mind and speed up the process of rewiring your brain, until your goal has become a part of you. The more you feel as though you are already in possession of your goal, the faster your seed will germinate and grow.

Neuroscientists tell us that when we feel in harmony with an idea, the brain rewires itself, ready to project a new reality for us to experience in this world. The world is the equivalent of a projection screen (a blank canvas), hooked up to billions of individual human brains. The billions of brains operating all over the world are governed by our conscious and subconscious minds. It is our dreams, thoughts, feelings, ideas and desires which are impressed on the brain, and therefore in this body and therefore in reality. In other words, you can create new neural pathways in your brain which will wire and fire together (thoughts and emotions becoming in sync with each other), when you constantly imagine and feel as though you are in possession of your dream. Your mind, brain and body *must* act accordingly.

Obviously, you need to take action when aiming to improve your life and relationships, but your behaviour will reflect the neural pathways you have created in your brain. Most of us were not given this information about the gestation period at school or college, but this is the law of nature. A failure to integrate the law of gestation is what frustrates millions of people. Many people want to enhance their relationships but continue to use their minds and brains in such a way that they are at odds with the gestation period. Things take time to manifest.

The law of opposites

The reason I often ask my clients at my seminars to ask themselves questions regarding finding a solution to their challenges is that I have learned to appreciate the law of opposites, also referred to as the law of polarity. There are two sides to everything. You can look at a tragedy but, with clear-sightedness, see that some good can come from it. I thought the worst thing that had happened to me was becoming utterly addicted to drugs and alcohol in my teens; however this misfortune introduced me to recovery aged 21. As a result, my life has been a constant process of gaining greater self-awareness, something that would otherwise have been denied to me had I drifted through life without exploring my mind.

Where there is death, there is birth: a generation dies and a new generation replaces them. Whenever we ask ourselves a question the answer is always available in the realm of thought and imagination. *The answer is the opposite of the question.* We just have to access the answer, either through our own imagination or knowledge, or call upon others to assist us.

A physicist will be quick to agree that everything that has always existed and will ever exist in already here in the present. Energy cannot be created or destroyed; life constantly changes into different forms. This includes every single thought, idea and desire that has ever been realized or has yet to be realized. *The solution to every single problem already exists, but has not yet*

103

manifested itself. This does not mean that as a species we will solve all of humanity's problems in our lifetime. It is, in fact, hard work to access un-manifested formula to life's challenges, which is why we celebrate when we have breakthroughs. Thoughts and ideas are not excluded from the fact that everything that ever was or ever will be is here. This might seem 'out there', but if you take your time to reread this chapter and this section on the law of opposites and interview physicists, this will become clearer.

For example, the theory of relativity existed, say, 20,000 years ago; it just took Albert Einstein to become aware of it in the twentieth century. His theory of relativity was lying dormant in the field of thought (keep in mind that we do not know exactly where thoughts 'reside' but we know that they are most certainly utilized by the human brain), beyond space and time, until he penetrated his brain and mind and drew upon higher thoughts and ideas. The formula to create a smartphone was available 5,000 years ago, again lying dormant in the field of thought, but it took Steve Jobs and his team to become aware of the smartphone formula in the 2000s. Humanity had to wait until 1903 for the first successful fixed-wing powered air flight, thanks to the Wright brothers. The formula to fly in the air was available during the Roman Empire, but we had to wait for the Wright brothers to draw upon their thoughts and imagination until they had their first successful flight. They were at the right place, at the right time, with the exact conditions necessary to create the first flight. There had been countless previous failed attempts to do so before this, indicating that there was a collective desire among scientists to achieve this goal. Humanity was ready to begin flying in the air. Although the formula was available to fly 2,000 years ago, humanity was not ready for it.

With respect to asking yourself the right questions to gain the answers you need to move forward to have a good relationship with yourself and others, you might not be ready just yet. You may have to take what might appear to be detours before you arrive at the answer you were looking for. My life has had many zigzags, and on many occasions I thought I was going in the wrong direction, but I was actually progressing. For example, it took me almost 15 years in recovery for me to fully appreciate how to rewire my own brain and change my subconscious programming. I had to work multiple Twelve Step programmes (five in total over a 15-year period), deep grief work, visualization, retreats and listening to thousands of hours of affirmative audios to change my unconscious belief system. I asked the question, 'How can I be rid of my subconscious programming in my first year in recovery?' I asked another question, 'How can I meet my ideal partner?', in my first year in recovery, and had to take all sorts of actions necessary to prepare myself to meet her, let alone sustain a relationship. I had to wait five and half years to meet my partner after I asked that question. I needed to change myself before I met her. Answers to our questions do not always take as long as five or 15 years; sometimes we can access answers within days, weeks and months. It depends on our level of self-awareness. When you begin to ask yourself questions with respect to improving your relationships, remember that the answer already exists; you just have to resonate with the answer. And by the time you do resonate with the answer, you will have become the person who did not need to ask the question in the first place.

There are no 'small acts' in life

One of the great tragedies of the twentieth century was the First World War. While it is certainly true the balance of power among the European nations was perilously fragile in 1913–14, it was the 'small act' of a modest chauffeur, Leopold Lojka, which triggered what would become the most lethal war the world had yet known. How ironic that, in an era of almost absolute deference, and of stuffy social and economic class systems dominated by European monarchs, it was a working-class man's mistaken decision that altered the course of history so dramatically. For it was during a visit to Sarajevo by the heir to the throne of the Austro-Hungarian Empire – Archduke Franz Ferdinand – that his chauffeur, the afore-mentioned Lojka, took a wrong turn into a side street. Archduke Franz Ferdinand's murderer, Gavrilo Princip, who had taken part in a failed assassination plot earlier in the day, happened to be sitting in a café in the street when Lojka unexpectedly drove towards him. Princip, a 19-year-old Bosnian Serb member of Young Bosnia, recognized Archduke Franz Ferdinand and shot and killed him. Because of a complex web of alliances, this became the spark of the First World War.

If we study history, we will find hundreds of examples of perceived 'small acts' which changed the course of history. Let us consider our own lives. Think of the perceived small acts which have changed your life. What if your parents hadn't met? What would have happened to you if you had gone to a different school or had never met your spouse/partner?

The truth is all actions are significant. The next time you procrastinate about putting five to ten minutes aside every morning and evening to visualize your goal, or to continue practising your recovery programmes, or attend a workshop or retreat, remember that such acts will accumulate over the days, weeks and months. Your 'small acts' will change your life.

Stay focused

The author Raymond Holliwell wrote: 'The mind is creating continually like fertile soil. Nature does not differentiate between the seed of a weed and that of a flower.' In other words, if you continue to allow yourself to be distracted and permit limiting beliefs, thoughts and emotions to germinate in your mind and brain, you will continue getting the same results. 'Energy flows where attention goes,' as the expression goes.

Now that you have your primary goal in mind, the challenge is to stay focused. Uncomfortable and perhaps even distressing emotions may arise if you are seriously stretching yourself and breaking through your comfort zone. This is why it is essential to have a team supporting you, at the very least one person you can regularly check in with and discuss your progress regarding your goal. Perseverance and some sort of meditation practice will keep you in good stead with respect to staying focused. There may be detours and perhaps you feel as though you are not advancing, but remember that your results will always reflect what progress has been made. Some goals take longer to manifest. Keep in mind that everything in this world has a gestation period. A seed takes time before it germinates. My experience is that, if you really want something, it will be on your mind most of the time.

The power of making a commitment

One of the biggest stumbling blocks I have observed over the years which hampers people's chances of creating and improving healthy relationships is because they have not understood the power of making a commitment. Essentially, a commitment follows a decision. We do not know what the future holds, but we decide to commit, nonetheless, after we have made a decision to do so.

Here is a personal example. I learned what the power of making a commitment can really do aged 21. I was a few days clean and sober, and I made a commitment to serve tea for an entire year at my local support group; I took on a tea commitment. By doing so, I was demonstrating to myself that I was capable of making a decision to do so and committing to my decision. I therefore begun to trust myself; I developed a bit more belief in myself. More importantly, I developed the habit of sticking to a commitment, which therefore spilled into other areas of my life. Within a year, I became a reliable person. People called on me to be of service and trusted in me to deliver. This was a huge contrast from my 21-year-old self who turned up at a recovery meeting, one day sober, with a reputation of being unreliable and 'flaky'. Over the years, I have enjoyed the power of making commitments to myself and others and seeing them through. There have been rare occasions in the last 15 years when I have not been able to fulfil on commitments due to emergencies, but I have found a way to make up for it by finding creative ways to direct my attention to serve my community in a different way.

There is incredible power in being committed to a relationship, a project or a goal. Something shifts in us, and we grow as a person. It was Ralph Waldo Emerson who said, 'Once you make a decision, the universe conspires to make it happen,' by which he meant that the right people and opportunities will be attracted to us to help us fulfil our commitments. How committed are you to heal your relationships and succeed in your life? All you have to do is make a decision to commit and the rest will fall into place.

Learning to reward yourself

Every time you achieve a goal or make a milestone in your recovery and personal growth, learning to reward yourself will create a deep imprint in your brain and body. You will be conditioning yourself to continue to expand your life and will become accustomed to receiving a reward for doing so. In other words, you can train yourself to feel good for taking action. As a result, you will create an incentive to enlarge your life, which will in turn inspire you to take action. Your self-belief and confidence will rise.

The difficulty for many people is that they have forgotten how to celebrate and reward themselves. There are all sorts of ways to reward ourselves. We can create subtle rewards or be extravagant. We can decide how we reward our achievements. This is a good time to put some time aside to think of creative ways to reward yourself. What can you do the next time you accomplish a goal and make progress in your life? The possibilities are endless.

The healing power of laughter

Almost all of us love to laugh and enjoy a good comedy show. Laughter brings us into harmony with joy. It reduces stress, eliminates anxiety and diminishes fear. We can transcend our regrets and sorrows thanks to the healing power of laughter. We all have different sense of humour: some of us like dark humour (think of Sacha Baron Cohen winding up a disgruntled, angry politician, an uncut Richard Pryor stand-up show, or Ricky Gervais in *The Office*), while some prefer family-friendly humour (think of Will Ferrell or shows like *Seinfeld* and *Friends*). Laughter has got me through dark times in my teens and especially in my early recovery–it was the ideal antidote to fear and bewilderment.

In the *Journal of Neuroscience*, an article titled 'Social Laughter Triggers Endogenous Opioid Release in Humans', by Sandra Manninen and her colleagues, concludes that 'baseline level and modulation of the μ-opioid system by social laughter could be an important neurochemical mechanism reinforcing and maintaining social bonds between humans'. In other words, laughing with our family and friends releases endorphins in the opioid receptors in the human brain, and therefore produces 'feel-good emotions'. Laughter can have a similar effect to that of a powerful mind- and mood-altering drug.

Gratitude – a deep reservoir of abundance

For untreated addictive personalities, the idea of moderation is preposterous. When a person arrests her addiction, she can learn to appreciate simple pleasures. We need simple pleasures. They are life's gold dust – they provide a daily dose of delight. In my view, it is not possible to appreciate simple pleasures unless we understand and integrate moderation in our habits. To moderate comes with practice, perseverance and prudence.

My partner's mother, Betty, recently gave me a classic china tea set. After I have put time aside to pray and meditate, I get immense pleasure from having a hot cup of tea first thing in the morning while watching or listening to an inspirational programme. Before I retire at night, I enjoy a hot camomile tea to end the day. This is a simple pleasure, but incredibly satisfying.

A simple pleasure can be enjoying sipping a glass of cold fresh water when it's a hot sunny day, tasting a piece of chocolate or a sweet fruit after a delicious meal. Listening to sublime music or going for a walk can be incredibly therapeutic. I appreciate walking in the woods and being in harmony with nature. The vibrational frequency of the trees and plants always clears my mind and anchors me in the feeling of gratitude and abundance.

It is important to appreciate simple pleasures and the good things we already have, while working towards improving our lives. We can even be grateful for our goals and the wonderful works of our imagination. We can be grateful that we have the mental faculties to create loving relationships and enhance our professional lives. Deep within us is an abundant reservoir of things we can appreciate. It is just a matter of our perception, our attention and a willingness to cultivate gratitude.

Write down 30 things which you are grateful for and share them with someone you love. It is worth doing this at least once a month, ideally once a week. Think of at least one thing every day you appreciate and emotionally connect with your expression of gratitude. You might find that such an attitude of appreciation will enhance your enthusiasm to participate in life in a more effective and meaningful way.

Deep inspiration

When we were children, it was easier to be in awe of everyday experiences. Seeing a bird take off in the air or watching a cat chasing a piece of string was amazing to my four-year-old self. I remember being amazed how my parents could drive a car. I was in awe of people who I believed lived in my parents' 'television box' – before the science of how a television works was explained to me. Even then, I was star struck by pop and movie stars.

As an adult, it has become harder for me to be in awe due to my mental conditioning. However, listening to music through an excellent sound system, at the appropriate volume, without distraction, is an easy way to be in awe. Travelling to new locations can bring a sense of wonder. Looking at a mountain or being out at sea can help me to rekindle deep reverence for the present moment. I can occasionally be in awe by listening to an inspirational story of recovery at a support group or at a convention. Being in awe often occurs when we are inspired and have experienced something which excites our inner child. Spiritual experiences and spiritual awakenings can certainly activate awe-inspiring moments of love and joy.

I have written a guided visualization meditation script for you to say out loud, record and play back to yourself. The purpose of this guided meditation is to assist you to expand your imagination, enhance your vision, and emotionally and physically connect with your primary goal. Play this both in the morning and evening for at least 90 days. After a while, you will not need to use this scripted meditation. The most important element in this guided visualization is to emotionally connect with your imagination.

Guided visualization meditation

Close your eyes.

Take a deep breath.

Now breathe in for four seconds, hold your breath for four seconds, and breathe out for four seconds.

Be aware that your body is breathing, and feel the breath enter and leave your body. Feel your stomach, as you breathe deeply in the present moment.

(*Pause for 20 seconds.*)

Continue to be mindful of the breath. Feel the breath flow in and out of your body, and relax.

(*Pause for 20 seconds.*)

It's important to relax, and so take a deep breath.

Now repeat out loud in the present tense your primary goal. Charge these words with enthusiasm and repeat your statement out loud five times.

Now take a deep breath.

Repeat your statement out loud again, but this time see yourself living your goal. See yourself clearly in this image.

(*Pause for 20 seconds.*)

Take three deep breaths.

See the colours brighten in your vision. Be aware of what you're wearing, your body posture and your chosen environment. There is no need to force this vision. Relax and take a deep breath. The more relaxed you are, the easier it will be to see your primary goal. So take a deep breath and bathe yourself in your dream reality.

(*Pause for 20 seconds.*)

Now take a deep breath and go deeper into relaxation.

Now sink deeply into the feeling as though you have already manifested your primary goal. In other words, imagine what it would feel like for this precious vision of yours to be a reality on the physical plane.

(*Pause for 20 seconds.*)

Feel your dream deeply and let your body connect with your vision. See and feel your vision as a matter of fact, right now, in the present. Let yourself relax.

(*Pause for 20 seconds.*)

Permit yourself to enjoy seeing and feeling your dream. This is truly a wonderful dream.

(*Pause for 20 seconds.*)

Take three deep breaths and begin to give thanks to the universe or life for your vision. Thank your mind and brain for the gift of being able to create your own environment. Sink deeply into the feeling of gratitude.

(*Pause for 20 seconds.*)

Continue to feel and believe your vision is a fact, and thank life for this fact, knowing that by doing so you are rewiring your brain and reprogramming your body.

Now take a deep breath and go deeper into relaxation. Now say your statement out loud and continue to charge your statement with gratitude and enthusiasm.

Take a deep breath and open your eyes.

End recording.

7

Limitations can spark creativity

If you are continually judging and criticizing yourself while trying to be kind to others, you are drawing artificial boundaries and distinctions that only lead to feelings of separation and isolation.

Kristin Neff

Frank Lloyd Wright once said: 'The human race built most nobly when limitations were greatest, and therefore where most was required of imagination in order to build it all. Limitations seem to have always been the best friends of architecture.' For years, I viewed my problems as some sort of curse, and I most definitely took it personally if things didn't go 'my way'. The fact is, I am always going to have problems to solve. There is no escaping this. I enjoy creating new goals, and so I expect to have to work through new challenges. I no longer expect 'something for nothing'. Such vicissitudes, when met with a positive attitude, help me to grow. Every time I solve a problem or successfully tackle a challenge, I know that I am consciously rewiring my brain, becoming a little bit smarter and emotionally stronger. It is these challenges which force me to access meditation and to use my imagination. They also compel me to ask for help and reach out to my fellow human beings. Rather than seeing problems as a curse, I have trained my mind to recognize that there can be a respect for the process of figuring out how to face difficulty. I do not always feel optimistic about problem solving; it often depends on simple contributory factors such as whether I have had enough sleep and eaten well.

Let us consider Frank Lloyd Wright's statement that humanity has always performed at a higher level under serious limitations. We can meditate on how humankind learned to create fire, dwellings to live in and ships to cross the oceans. When the entire world was convinced that humankind would never fly in powered machines, there came an astounding breakthrough which meant that we could indeed travel through the air.

Consider how many people died from addiction, eating disorders and mental illness before the twentieth century. Alcoholics, drug addicts, anorexics and bulimics were left to die lonely deaths or were locked away. Apart from the Washingtonian movement in the nineteenth century, which fizzled out after a few years, drug addicts and alcoholics were considered hopeless cases until Alcoholics Anonymous was founded in the USA on 10 June 1935. The AA movement paved the way for dozens of Twelve Step fellowships addressing addictions and dysfunctional behaviour and indirectly created the addiction/recovery movement worldwide. Such recovery movements have arrested addiction and put millions of people's illnesses into remission.

If we think about Frank Lloyd Wright's statement and emotionally internalize it, we can see that our greatest challenges have often transformed us into stronger and wiser human beings. Even those of us who have found it hard to create safe, non-shaming and trusting relationships can use this as a springboard to becoming the person we wish to be and to attract the people we truly want in our lives. I myself have been able to do a 180-degree turnaround, from being a dysfunctional person who attracted toxic relationships to discovering my true self who attracted authentic and meaningful ones. In hindsight, my suffering and emotional pain were my secret treasure trove. If I can do this, then so can you.

Limitations help us to stretch ourselves so that we can evolve

If we want to be in a healthy loving relationship, we have to be kind and loving towards ourselves and others. If we want to attract an ideal long-term partner with appealing character traits, we, too, have to demonstrate such appealing characteristics so that we can match their vibrational frequency. We have to be capable of *being* in a loving romantic relationship, and have the skillset properly in place, before we can attract a partner, let alone sustain and evolve in such a relationship. If we want to attract prosperous business associates and competent professionals to work with, we have to bring something to the table. If we want to expand in our careers and have a vision of ourselves progressing, we have to become the person capable of achieving this vision. We have to stretch ourselves so that we can match the higher vision we have of ourselves. We have to *be* the person we want to attract.

I have had to come out of my comfort zone hundreds of times in order to grow as a person and match my ideal vision of myself. It has not been easy, but persistence eventually brings untold rewards. My recovery has been a process of working on and improving different areas in my life. I have learned that we can only change one habit at a time. Once a habit is firmly fixed in our brains and bodies, we can move on to develop a new habit. One new habit can change our lives in the most surprising ways. The problem is many people attempt to address all of their habits at once, which subsequently leads to them feeling overwhelmed and despondency setting in. The key contributing factor in overcoming our limitations (which are a composed of our thoughts, feelings and actions) is to simplify the process: addressing one habit at a time, one day at a time, and discussing our progress with an understanding person as often as we can.

HALT: hungry, angry, lonely and tired

There is an acronym often quoted in recovery circles: HALT, meaning 'hungry, angry, lonely and tired'. It is important to be mindful of these common basic human conditions and to act accordingly. We are much less likely to feel overwhelmed by our challenges if we are looking after our most basic needs. It can be easy to skip eating in the workplace as a result of feeling that we have too much work to get through. We can often ignore angry feelings towards another person or a feeling of isolation. There is usually a price to pay for this.

Feeling tired is another state which can stifle our creativity and compel us to make unnecessary mistakes. The 14th Dalai Lama once said, 'Sleep is the best meditation', and I am inclined to agree with him. Although there is still a widely accepted view that we should sleep for the shortest time possible if we are make the most of a 24-hour day, most human beings tend to perform infinitely better when they have had a good night's sleep and enjoyed a good REM cycle (usually seven to eight hours). For those of us who enjoy lucid dreaming and the benefits of finding answers to our problems which this can provide, a good night's sleep is essential. Whether we choose to get enough hours' sleep to perform better in our lives or to access buried memories and creative thoughts, we can learn to appreciate the wonderful benefits of this sacred time.

It took me many years to get to bed at a reasonable time due to having previously worked as a DJ in nightclubs. I now appreciate the joy of waking up and retiring early. I have found that if I get enough sleep, I am less likely to be triggered by other people's behaviour.

It takes courage to ask for help

By answering all the questions in this book and discussing your answers with a non-shaming action partner, mentor or a trusted friend, you will have reached a better understanding of where you are and what you need to do to improve in certain areas of your life. You will have a goal in mind and understand the process of visualization, meditation and how to use your imagination to change your life for the better. The good news is that we can work on a particular area in our lives to achieve improvement until such a practice becomes a fixed habit. Please do not feel overwhelmed by this. I, too, am still working on improving my life and will continue to do so until I draw my last breath. Self-improvement is a lifelong process.

The fear of being shamed privately or publicly is what stops many people from reaching out and asking for help. Some people prefer to suffer alone in silent desperation, rather than taking a risk and reaching out for help. It takes courage to ask for help. It is not a weakness. It is a sign of humility and strength. Make asking for help your primary habit; it will lead you to answers about how to better serve yourself and therefore others.

I learned how to ask for help when I attended my first Twelve Step meeting aged 19 and admitted to a group of 50 drug addicts and alcoholics that I was addicted to alcohol and mind- and mood-altering drugs. I was terribly nervous leading up to the meeting, but I desperately needed help. I was willing to make myself vulnerable in order to save my life. Throughout my recovery and personal development, I have had to ask for assistance. If you take anything away from this book, I ask you to seriously consider how regularly asking for help or seeking counsel can fundamentally change your life.

I wish you the very best.

Christopher

References

Chapter 1

James Allen, *As a Man Thinketh* (CreateSpace Independent Publishing Platform, 2013).

Barbara Mariposa and Christopher Dines, *The Kindness Habit: Transforming our Relationship to Addictive Behaviours* (Riverbank Books, 2016).

Maria Montessori, *The Absorbent Mind* (BNN Publishing, 2009).

Chapter 2

John Bradshaw, *Healing the Shame That Binds You*, rev. edn (Health Communcations, 2006).

Kelly McNelis, *Your Messy Brilliance: 7 Tools for the Perfectly Imperfect Woman* (Enrealment Press, 2017).

Research by Dr Keon West:
see https://www.gold.ac.uk/news/naked-and-unashamed/

Chapter 3

Deepak Chora and Rudolph E. Tanzi, *The Healing Self: Supercharge Your Immune System and Stay Well for Life* (Rider, 2018).

Deepak Chora and Rudolph E. Tanzi, *Super Brain: Unleashing the Explosive Power of Your Mind to Maximize Health, Happiness and Spiritual Well-Being* (Rider, 2013).

Deepak Chora and Rudolph E. Tanzi, *Super Genes; The Hidden Key to Total Well-being* (Rider, 2013).

Eckhart Tolle, *The Power of Now: A Guide to Spiritual Enlightenment* (Yellow Kite, 2016).

Barbara Mariposa and Christopher Dines, *The Kindness Habit: Transforming our Relationship to Addictive Behaviours* (Riverbank Books, 2016).

Mark Williams, John Teasdale, Zindel Segal and Jon Kabat Zinn, *The Mindful Way through Depression: Freeing yourself from Chronic Unhappiness* (Guilford Press, 2007).

Chapter 4

Shawn Meghan Burn, quoted at
https://bpdfamily.com/content/codependency-codependent-relationships

Christopher Dines, *Drug Addiction Recovery* (Sheldon Press, 2019).

Christopher Dines, *Mindfulness Burnout Prevention: An 8-Week Course for Professionals* (La Petite Fleur, 2015).

Pia Mellody, *Facing Codependence: What It Is, Where It Comes from, How It Sabotages Our Lives* (HarperOne, 2002).

Chapter 6

Christopher Dines, 'Super Brain, Super Genes and Alzheimer's – Dr. Rudy Tanzi Interview (Part One)',
https://www.huffingtonpost.co.uk/christopher-dines/super-brain-super-genes-a_b_12521256.html

Christopher Dines, *The Mystery of Belief; How to Manifest Your Dreams* (La Petite Fleur Publishing, 2013).

Napoleon Hill, *Think & Grow Rich; The Original Version, Restored and Revised* (Mindpower Press; Revised edition, 2015).

Raymond Holliwell, *Working With the Law; 11 Truth Principles for Successful Living* (DeVorss & Company; Rev. Ed edition, 2005).

Sandra Manninen and others, 'Social Laughter Triggers Endogenous Opioid Release in Humans', *Journal of Neuroscience* 37:25 (June 2017): 6125–31.

Dan Siegel, 'How You Can Change Your Brain',
https://www.psychalive.org/how-you-can-change-your-brain/

Brooklyn Storme, 'An Introduction to the Neuroscience behind Creating Your Reality',
https://psychcentral.com/blog/an-introduction-to-the-neuroscience-behind-creating-your-reality/

Ben Wilson and others, *Alcoholics Anonymous: The Story of How Many Thousands of Men and Women Have Recovered from Alcoholism*, rev. edn (AA, 1976).

Index